Foundations of Health
The Liver and Digestion Herbal

Christopher Hobbs

Foreword by Bernard Jensen

Look for other books available from

Botanica Press

by **Christopher Hobbs**

In book stores and natural food stores throughout the U.S.

The Herbs and Health Series:

Echinacea! The Immune Herb
Usnea: The Herbal Antibiotic
Medicinal Mushrooms
Natural Liver Therapy
Vitex: The Women's Herb
Milk Thistle: The Liver Herb
Ginkgo, Elixir of Youth
Medicinal Plant Constituents,
  Symbols of Healing Energy

Copyright September, 1992
by Christopher Hobbs

Michael Miovic, editor
Beth Baugh, copy editor
Mark Johnson, cartoons, illustrations
Plant illustrations copyright, Donna Cehrs, Sept. 1992
Yellow Dock illustration by Rose Ducale
Anatomy illustration by Francine Martin

Botanica Press
Box 742
Capitola, CA

*This book is dedicated to my mother and father,
and to my great teachers, Paul C. Bragg
and Vivekananda.*

Our commitment
We at Botanica Press are dedicated in our personal and professional lives
to environmental awareness.
We are strongly committed to recycling, and we gladly contribute a
portion of our profits to the Nature
Conservancy and other conservation groups
*This book is printed on recycled paper with a minimum of
10% post-consumer waste, and the entire text is printed using non-toxic
soy-based ink

The information in this book is meant to be for educational purposes, indicating recent laboratory and clinical work as well as a summary of the history of use of traditional herbal remedies and not as a recommendation as a cure for any disease. If a serious health imbalance is present, the author recommends seeking the advice of a qualified holistic health practitioner.

Table of Contents

Chapter 4

**Probiotics, Human Body Ecology
and Intestinal Gardening**

Chapter 5

Herbal Therapy

Foreword

It was a great pleasure and an honor on my part to read the original manuscript of this book from Christopher Hobbs.

Is there anything in life that we would like to have more than good health? Without health, how can we meet the challenges of the day? How can we be fit for what is coming tomorrow? So many people today realize that self-care has to be instituted in our homes; that our homes should be wellness centers, and we have to start right at the kitchen table to take care of ourselves and our children.

It is important to know how to take care of ourselves so that we are free of the pains, aches, and acute ailments that may ultimately develop into chronic and degenerative diseases. We stop this process in the beginning when we realize, as we see in *Foundation of Health*, that these develop when our digestion is not in good order. In creating health, digestion is the first thing to consider. We cannot expect the tissues in our body to remain in a state of optimum health unless we have an evolved way of living, which springs from knowledge and wisdom.

It is my experience, that in cleansing and taking care of the body, the four channels of elimination—the kidney, the bowels, the bronchial tree and lungs, and the skin—are most important. When these are working well and are in a state of purity with no underlying toxicity to act as sources of infection, then we are ready to enjoy life to its fullest.

I have found that good health is very seldom felt by the average person in life. The medical profession tells us that 8 out of 10 people who say they feel well have a chronic disease. Is it possible that we could be walking around in a process of degeneration, never knowing what we are up against? The American Cancer Society tells us that it takes 20 years to develop a cancer. When a person has cancer, doctors are all too present, but I often wonder, where are they in the very beginning of the process? The best doctor is a preventative way of living. It's our lifestyle and what we do at the kitchen table. It's in our "dining room knowledge," in the food we put on our plate. This is the knowledge that should be spread among patients and doctors alike.

There are many ways of taking care of our digestion. We find that nutrition is probably the greatest art of salvation when it comes to keeping us well and fit for tomorrow than any other art that exists. Within 18 hours, that which comes into our body goes through the digestive tract and is set up to be delivered by our blood stream to every organ in the body. When every cell has been fed properly with perfectly digested foods, we find that the health of our tissues and organs, and of our whole body and mind, will be of the highest order possible.

The thing that I have always tried to work out in my teachings is to stress the importance of food in creating tissue of the highest integrity possible. This goes back to the soil, back to the plants, and knowing how to buy and prepare our foods properly. We also have to recognize that variety is important.

I feel that anyone who is on the path of health should use this book of knowledge, which will give them a complete guide to the Foundations of Health, including dietary and herbal recommendations for taking care of various health problems.

My prayer has been for those people who are seeking abundant health to have good literature and people with good hearts who want to serve. It is with great pleasure, then, that I recommend *Foundations of Health* very sincerely.

With all best wishes,

Bernard Jensen

Note from the Author

This book is written to share over 20 years of experience and experimentation with diet and digestion. In this time, I have tried every diet imaginable–including the "McDonalds" diet (attacked by the Big Mac), the Kentucky Fried Chicken diet, a fruitarian diet, a raw foods diet, a macrobiotic diet, and many other types of diets as well. Being immoderate by nature, it has taken me many years to reach a balance. However, at last I feel that I have reached a personal balance–though diet by nature must change constantly with the seasons, the type of work one is doing, and other needs.

Over 20 years ago I had hepatitis twice. My digestion and liver were in terrible shape from excessive social drinking and other abusive habits. After a few years of serious digestive problems that lead to improper absorption of nutrients and a weakened immune system, I discovered the healing power of herbs, including milk thistle, which I eventually wrote about in my booklet *Milk Thistle, The Liver Herb*. This, along with a radically different view of diet and health that I received from my teacher, Paul C. Bragg, put me firmly on my own healing journey–a lifelong path that continues today.

Special thanks to Beth, who was untiring in her efforts to make this book as perfect as humanly possible and to Michael Miovic, our super-editor, who helped make the words flow.

Christopher Hobbs

Introduction

Many practitioners of natural healing emphasize that digestion is truly the foundation of health. Digestion is our power center—the translator and regulator of our physical energy. It gives the body energy to live and grow, and is intimately involved in maintaining all of the bodily processes and systems. However, digestion also provides the energy for many human activities that are not usually associated with food and eating—such as the mental energy of a scientist or thinker, and the emotional and creative energy of an artist or musician. So, ultimately, the motive force or energy that fuels all life activities derives from the basic process called digestion.

But what exactly does digestion consist of? At root, digestion is made up of two opposite yet complementary physical processes: assimilation and elimination. These two processes are basic to all life forms, from one-celled organisms to human beings. All creatures need to assimilate nutrients that are necessary to maintain life processes and functions, and they need to eliminate wastes that are unnecessary or even toxic. When the processes of assimilation and elimination work smoothly and are in balance in an organism it is healthy. When either process is excessive or deficient, sooner or later that organism becomes unhealthy, or diseased. Thus, in a very real sense, the old adage that we are what we eat is quite true—though a more accurate way to state this idea would be to say that

1

we are what we assimilate. (I once heard someone go one step further and state, "We are what we don't eliminate." Thus perhaps
the best thing to say is, "We are what we assimilate and don't eliminate"! Alas, in today's world, we are continually assimilating and
not eliminating environmental toxins and contaminants that endan-
ger our health.)

Interestingly, the processes of assimilation and elimination are
not confined to just the physical realm; they operate at the emotional, mental, and even spiritual levels of our beings as well. Although the scope of this book does not allow for a full discussion of
assimilation and elimination in this extended sense, I will give a few
examples that illustrate the general concept. Take emotional nourishment, for instance: we all need to receive (or assimilate) expressions of love and caring such as attention, kind words, hugs, and so
on; and we all need to eliminate negative emotions through reflection, taking action, crying, laughing, and other methods.

At the mental level, we get nourishment from many sources,
including conversations, books, movies, puzzles, problems, our
own thoughts and experiences, etc. We have to "digest" new ideas
and information in order to understand them, and then we have to
eliminate old ideas and concepts that no longer fit our revised view
of reality. And finally, at the spiritual level, we have to assimilate
and digest all of the experiences we have in life and eliminate our
attachments to the physical, emotional, and mental levels of existence. As we do this, slowly we learn to live more and more in our
true spiritual natures. Eventually, a person who has fully assimilated
the spiritual lessons of life may even eliminate attachment to the
physical body altogether, as can be seen in the examples of highly
advanced souls such as Ramakrishna, Vivekananda, Ramana

Maharshi, and the saints and spiritual masters of many other cultures and religious traditions.

As I have said above, this book will focus primarily on the physical aspects of digestion, because these have a very direct and immediate effect on our general sense of health and well-being.

Although it is certainly true that mind and body interact with and affect each other, there is simply not room in this work to address all of these issues in their entirety. However, I will discuss psychological techniques for promoting health and happiness, but mostly I will explore natural dietary and herbal means for treating a variety of common digestion-related disorders, including gas, nausea, constipation, obesity, emotional imbalances, addictions, lowered vitality, and decreased immune strength. If you are interested in complementing the information presented in this book with further information about psychological and spiritual methods for promoting greater well-being, see the list of recommended reading on pages 290 and 291.

Finally, please note that this book is divided into three major sections:

I. **Background Information** This section explains how digestion works according to both modern science and Traditional Chinese Medicine.

II. **Natural Therapies** This section gives information and recommendations regarding various natural methods of treating digestive disorders and improving general health.

III. **Herbal** This section contains detailed information about the properties and uses of important digestive herbs.

Chapter 1

The Digestive System

Before we jump right into discussing various natural methods for improving digestion, it would be useful first to have a general idea of what the digestive system is and does—that is, what its major organs are and how they function. Perhaps the best place to begin this overview of the digestive system is with food, since the whole purpose of the digestive system is to extract the energy stored in food.

Western Viewpoint

In scientific terms, all food-energy is chemical energy. That is, it comes from the energy stored in the chemical bonds between the elements that make up the various foods we eat. In general, all foods are composed of three broad classes of chemical compounds: carbohydrates, proteins, and fats (or lipids). The details about the chemical structures of these compounds don't mean much unless you have a fairly good knowledge of chemistry. However, almost everyone these days knows something about which foods contain these different classes of compounds and how much of each food one should eat.

Carbohydrates are the broadest class of chemical compounds in food. They include all forms of sugar, starch, and cellulose. Thus carbohydrates are found in all foods that contain either synthetic or naturally occurring sugars; in starch-containing

4

foods such as corn, potatoes, wheat, and rice; and in all vegetables, since plants are made mostly of cellulose. Interestingly, however, the human body cannot digest cellulose very well; therefore it extracts only a little energy from this type of carbohydrate.

Proteins, as most people know, are energy-rich substances that are found in foods such as meat, seeds and nuts, milk, eggs, and all types of beans. These foods are eaten to increase strength and endurance.

Finally, fats are found in foods such as butter, margarine, lard, cheese, animal fat, and cooking oils. Fats are also rich sources of energy, but they tend to be stored in the body much longer than proteins, which is why they can cause excessive weight-gain.

Now carbohydrates, proteins, and fats are all fairly large molecules built out of long chains of various types of atoms. *Digestion* is nothing more and nothing less than the process of breaking these large molecules down into smaller "pieces" that the body can absorb. As it turns out, the body has two major ways of breaking down food: mechanical methods and chemical methods.

Mechanical methods of digestion include chewing, which happens in the mouth, and mixing and churning, which happen in the stomach and intestines. These methods all increase the *surface area* of food exposed to gastric juices.

Chemical digestion, on the other hand, is carried out by the digestive juices themselves and actually alters the chemical structure of food. This sort of digestion is done by chemical substances such as hydrochloric acid (in the stomach); bile (made in the liver); and numerous types of *enzymes*, each of which is designed to break down a specific type of compound. (For your information, any time a substance ends in the letters -ase, it is an enzyme. You may find this helpful as you read the rest of this chapter.) Thus, it is the chemical methods of digestion that ultimately produce the tiny nutritional "pieces" the body can absorb and use for energy.

Hopefully the preceding explanation gives you some idea of what the digestive system as a whole is trying to accomplish. To give you a clearer picture of the steps of the process and where each step occurs in the body, we will now follow a meal from the moment it is ingested through one end of the alimentary canal until it is finally excreted out the other.

When food enters the mouth, it is chewed by the teeth and mixed with saliva, which contains an enzyme that starts to break down carbohydrates. After the food has been chewed and formed loosely into a little ball called a *bolus*, it is swallowed and passes through the esophagus to reach the stomach. In the stomach, the bolus is churned and mixed with gastric juices, creating a thin liquid called *chyme*. The process of breaking down protein begins in the stomach and continues in the small intestine, where the chyme is acted on by pancreatic, liver, and other enzymes. In the small intestine, about 90% of simple sugars, fats, and proteins are absorbed into the bloodstream (the other 10% are absorbed either before, in the stomach, or after, in the large intestine).

Any food residues that are not broken down and absorbed in the small intestine (mainly cellulose and other insoluble fibers) are passed on to the large intestine, where they are acted on by various microorganisms, mostly bacteria. Because of this activity, the body is able to extract some energy and nutrition from plant fibers that would otherwise be indigestible. In the large intestine, the feces are formed from the indigestible portions of food and other bodily wastes, and finally the feces are excreted via the anus. All the while, the food bolus, and later the feces, are moved along by the contractions of the smooth muscle of the digestive tract, a process called *peristalsis.*

That is a general outline of the digestive process. Now let's take a closer look at some of the key steps and organs involved in the process.

The First Step of Digestion: The Brain

An important first step of digestion that most of us overlook in daily life is the brain, or mind, and nervous system. We usually think of digestion beginning in the mouth and progressing downward, but really the whole process begins even higher in the body, in the brain. To prove this to yourself, imagine a nice juicy tofu burger—or, if you prefer, imagine something more "meaty." But whatever your favorite food is, imagine it now. Can you feel the saliva starting to flow in your mouth? Can you hear a rumbling sound in your gut? If you imagine your chosen food well enough, you probably will. This is because by imagining a delicious meal, you are actually causing your brain to prepare your body for that meal. And if you were now to go ahead and really eat your juicy burger, you would probably have excellent digestion, because your digestive tract has been "prepped" for the job.

The mental component of digestion is rarely discussed. This is unfortunate, since it may be the single most significant factor in determining how effectively you extract vital nutrients from your food and how thoroughly you are able to eliminate the

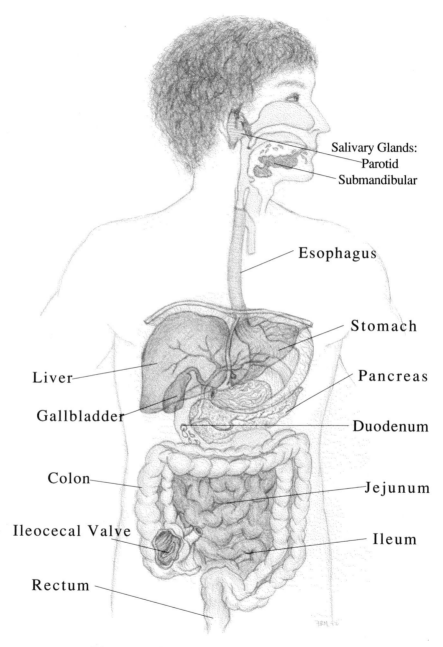

Fig. 1   The Human Digestive Tract

toxic by-products of digestion from your system. For instance, food that is beautifully prepared and presented will have a much better chance of being completely assimilated and later properly eliminated than food thrown together on the run. The atmosphere, both internal and external, in which you eat also makes a great difference. If you eat when feeling depressed, angry, or otherwise emotionally upset, your digestion will not be as good as when you eat in a pleasant ambience, and feel relaxed and peaceful. Likewise, your digestion and assimilation will be worse if you eat out of frustration or boredom than if you eat when truly hungry, as after refreshing physical activity.

The Mouth

In our usual way of thinking, digestion begins in the mouth, when food is chewed into small pieces and mixed with saliva. It is important to chew food thoroughly, so that it gets well mixed with this powerful digestive juice (see the sidebar for more information). When food is not well mixed with saliva, the stomach must work harder to churn it and produce more digestive enzymes to break it down. Also, when food is swallowed in large pieces, it may not even be completely digested by the time it reaches the colon—and thus the body can't extract all the useful nutrients from it. Many teachers of healthy living, including Paul Bragg and Michio Kushi, have emphasized the importance of thorough mastication.

Once food enters the stomach and moves on, you cannot say "a little more hydrochloric acid, if you please!" It is important to remember that food selection, presentation, and chewing are ways we can voluntarily affect the outcome of digestion.

The Digestive Power of Saliva

Saliva is produced in the mouth in response to the sight, smell, or taste of food. Saliva is composed mostly of water, which provides a medium that allows the flavoring agents in food to come into contact with the taste buds, thus enhancing the enjoyment of food. However, saliva also contains an important digestive enzyme called *amylase*, as well as *lysozyme*, an enzyme that kills pathogenic bacteria. Amylase begins the chemical digestion of carbohydrates. If carbohydrates are held in the mouth long enough, they begin to taste sweet. This indicates that the bonds between the sugars are being severed. You can notice this effect even with starches that initially don't taste sweet if you chew them long enough. Unfortunately, we usually swallow our food so quickly that only 3-5% of the carbohydrates can be reduced to disaccharides (small units that make up sugar molecules) in the mouth. The amylase does keep on working for up to 30 minutes in the stomach. However, because most simple sugars are absorbed in the small intestine, when starches are improperly chewed and mixed with amylase, some carbohydrates may make it all the way to the large intestine. This is undesirable, since bacteria can cause carbohydrates to ferment, creating gas. Thus, the bottom line here is, if you have trouble with gas, try chewing each bite of your food 30 or 40 times! Make sure it is well mixed with saliva before swallowing.

The Stomach

The stomach is situated just below the diaphragm. When the stomach is empty it is only the size of a large sausage. Yet it is able to stretch to the size of a large sac to hold big meals.

In the lining of the stomach (the mucosa) lie small pits, which are the gastric glands. These glands secrete *pepsinogen*, *hydrochloric acid*, *mucus*, and a substance called *intrinsic factor*. The pepsinogen is not an active gastric juice when it comes out of the gland. However, when it comes in contact with hydrochloric acid in the stomach, it turns into *pepsin*, which is the most important protein-digesting enzyme. Pepsin breaks large protein molecules into smaller units called *peptides* . Meanwhile, mucus forms a protective barrier that prevents pepsin and hydrochloric acid from harming the walls of the stomach. Nonetheless, sometimes this mucus thins out or fails to do its job, and a gastric ulcer results.

The stomach also produces *gastric lipase*, an enzyme that splits apart the butterfat molecules found in milk. This enzyme is more active in infants and children than in adults.

The stomach empties its contents into the upper small intestine (called the *duodenum*) a few hours after the food is eaten. Carbohydrates are the most quickly digested compounds in food, leaving the stomach in about three hours; proteins are next; and fats are the slowest to be digested. Thus, mixing fats with carbohydrates and proteins, as happens in stir-frying or deep-frying, can greatly slow the absorption, which may lead to painful gas. It may also allow irritating substances to come into contact with the walls of the intestine, and it may give toxic substances the chance to be absorbed.

Although the vast majority of nutrients are absorbed from the small intestine, a few things, such as salts, water, some drugs, and alcohol, can be absorbed in the stomach.

The Small Intestine

The small intestine is about 21 feet long and is divided into three parts: the upper section is called the *duodenum*; the middle part is the *jejunum*; and finally, the lower part is called the *ileum*. The duodenum is connected to the lower stomach through the pyloric valve, while the ileum is connected to the large intestine through the ileocecal valve.

Like the stomach, the small intestine is lined with mucous membranes that have pits which secrete various digestive substances. The walls of the small intestine are also lined with 4-5 million tiny finger-like projections called *microvilli*. These effectively expand the total surface area the small intestine has to absorb nutrients by many times. This accounts for why most carbohydrates, fats, and proteins are absorbed into the bloodstream in the small intestine.

Many enzymes are present in the small intestine to help digest carbohydrates, proteins, and fats. Some of these enzymes are produced in the small intestine, but many come from the liver and pancreas. The following table lists the major digestive enzymes that are active in the small intestine, their origins, and their functions.

The Large Intestine

The large intestine is about 5 feet long and averages 2.5 inches in diameter. It is divided into the cecum, colon, rectum, and anal canal (see figure 1). The colon is divided into the ascending, transverse, descending, and sigmoid sections.

During the period chyme is in the colon (3 to 10 hours), water is gradually absorbed from it back into the body, making the mass more solid. Dead bacteria, bacterial by-products, undigested insoluble fibers, mucus, and dead cells from the walls of the intestines all accumulate and are mixed with the solidified chyme to become feces, which are then passed out of the body.

Table 1
Major Digestive Enzymes in the Small Intestine

Enzyme	Source	Function
*Fat Digestion		
Bile	liver	emulsifies (or breaks apart) fats into droplets
Bile salts	liver	breaks fat droplets into even smaller droplets
Pancreatic lipase	pancreas	breaks apart every fat molecule into fatty acids, glycerol, and glycerides, which are absorbed
*Carbohydrate Digestion		
Pancreatic amylase	pancreas	breaks down carbohydrates into maltose
Maltase	small intestine	splits maltose into two molecules of glucose
Sucrase	small intestine	breaks sucrose into a molecule of glucose and one of fructose
Lactase	small intestine	breaks lactose into a molecule of glucose and one of galactose
*Protein Digestion		
Trypsin	pancreas	splits any intact proteins (that escaped stomach peptase) into smaller chains of amino acids called peptones and proteoses, which it in turn breaks into dipeptides (units of two amino acids) and even single amino acid units
Chymotripsin	small intestine	similar activity to trypsin
Carboxy-peptidase	small intestine	breaks partly digested amino acid chains into single amino acid units
Erpepsin	small intestine	a group of enzymes that reduces any final dipeptides into single amino acids

The large intestine also contains a large number of beneficial bacteria, which are collectively called the *intestinal microflora*, or IM for short.   The IM is remarkable because it produces B vitamins and vitamin K, and it ferments undigested insoluble fiber to produce compounds that are absorbed by the cells in the lining of the colon. This may be an important source of energy for the cells of the colon and thus save the body valuable energy overall.   Finally, the IM breaks down any undigested proteins and even amino acids into substances that contribute to the odor of feces. We will return to the IM in depth in Chapter 4.

The Digestive System in Traditional Chinese Medicine

Ancient Chinese doctors did not have the detailed anatomical and physiological knowledge of the body that modern science has developed. However, they were very acute observers of health and illness, and they developed methods of diagnosis and treatment that are remarkably coherent and effective given the limitations under which these doctors were working. The conclusions Chinese doctors reached, based on an unbroken tradition of thousands of years of observation and clinical experimentation, have been collected and integrated to form the system of medicine now known as Traditional Chinese Medicine (TCM). TCM is still widely accepted and practiced in China today, and thanks to the successes acupuncture has demonstrated in alleviating chronic pain, it is now gaining acceptance in Western countries, too. Open-minded doctors working in TCM and Western scientific medicine agree that both traditions have much to offer each other, and that the medicine of the future will probably be based on a scientific understanding of some of the subtler relations between mind and body which TCM has long recognized.

Now the concept of the digestive system in TCM is in most ways similar to the way Western science understands this group of organs. TCM recognizes the existence of the liver, stomach, gallbladder, small intestine, and large intestine.

The only major difference in TCM's understanding of the digestive process is the function it ascribes to the spleen. According to Western anatomy and physiology, the spleen contains many lymph cells, is involved in certain immune functions, breaks down old or damaged red blood cells, and stores and releases blood per the body's needs. In TCM, however, the spleen is primarily a digestive organ. Its main function is to control the whole process of extracting energy (or nutrition) from the foods that we eat.

All during this process, the spleen is transforming the food, distilling out the pure from the impure, and moving it upward

Original Qi

When we are born, we receive a gift of vitality from our ancestors, through our parents. This vitality is sometimes called "Original Qi." Throughout life, all of our organs and activities need a constant supply of energy and vitality. Much of this day to day energy is ideally supplied by the food we eat and the air we breathe. From the air, the lungs take out the "prana" (as it is called in Ayurveda) and from our food, the spleen separates the vitality inherent in it as well as other useful elements.

Therefore, the Chinese Spleen system is the foundation of much of our energy and vitality here on earth. It is the "central axis," as Maciocia (1989) calls it.

to the heart and lungs, where it becomes Qi and Blood.

Thus, in TCM the very core of the digestive system is considered to be the stomach/spleen "axis." Perhaps the best way for Westerners to think of the Chinese spleen is not as a physical organ, but rather as the set of processes which encompass various digestive functions of the small intestine and pancreas as well as other digestive organs.

The stomach is closely associated with the spleen and is said to control the transportation of food essences and give rise to the fluids in the body. Its job is to "rot and ripen" food and transmit the "impure residues" down to the small intestine, where the food is further transformed and its energy is extracted. "Clean" residues are absorbed into the body to give nutrition, and "dirty" residues are passed on to the large intestine, where useful moisture is separated out. What is left is waste and is eliminated as feces.

Organ System Relationships in TCM

Traditional Chinese Medicine recognizes five bodily systems, each of which is associated with one of the five primary elements in nature. Also, each of the principal internal organs is thought to be connected to an external part of the body which it affects, to an external anatomical part where the condition of the internal organ is reflected, and to an emotion and climatic condition. Table 2 summarizes these basic relationships.

Table 2
The Fundamental Relationship of TCM

Organ Systems	Element	Diag. Part	Affected Parts	Climate	Taste	Emotion
stomach/ spleen	earth	flesh, lips	mouth	moisture	sweet	self-pity
lungs/ colon	metal	nasal	skin/ cavities hair	dryness body	acrid	grief, despair
kidney/ bladder	water	ears	bones, head, hair, brain	coldness	salty	fear, anxiety
liver/ gallbladder	wood	eyes	tendons, nails, ligaments	wind	sour	anger
heart/ pericardium/ small intestine	fire	tongue	vascular system, complexion	heat	bitter	excite- ment, fright

Chapter 2

The Liver in Health and Illness

The Liver Means Life

In this chapter, I will place special emphasis on the liver. Other organs of digestion, such as the stomach, pancreas, and small intestine, play an important role in the process of digestion, but our liver is well worth a closer look because of its special role not only in digestion, but in a number of other vital bodily functions, such as energy storage, detoxification, and even as a secondary immune organ.

The liver is a remarkable organ and is largely unappreciated for the many vital functions it performs. It has been said that it is not called the *live-r* for nothing: it keeps us living. For instance, the liver is responsible for handling most of our energy needs. It takes raw materials from food (carbohydrates, fats, sugars, or proteins) and breaks these down into their basic components. Then it creates and stores glycogen (animal starch, which consists of long chains of sugars) for both immediate and long-term use as an energy source. Thus, if the liver is congested or diseased, it will not receive and send out enough blood, and one's energy level will suffer drastically. Thus, if you are experiencing a chronic lack of energy, especially after meals, it would be beneficial to focus on liver health.

The importance of keeping the liver open, healthy, and functioning smoothly is understood by doctors and herbalists

18

alike. The liver is the major organ of digestion and assimilation, helping to provide the nutrients that maintain health and repair diseased or damaged tissue. The liver also provides a vital function in helping to eliminate toxic wastes from the body. Unfortunately, however, liver disease is currently a common cause of death in this country—a tragic situation that could be prevented with proper dietary habits and natural liver therapy.

But why do so many people suffer from liver disease? There are several reasons. One is that the modern environment is full of stressful chemicals, such as lead from gasoline, countless food additives, preservatives, pesticides, herbicides, and many other new compounds. It is estimated that chemical companies, in their search for marketable compounds, produce hundreds of new chemicals every year. Since these compounds are completely new to the environment, we may not be able to adapt to them for thousands of years, so it is no wonder they can disrupt the delicate biochemistry of the body. For the liver this is especially significant because, among the internal organs, it is the liver that bears the brunt of many of these foreign compounds, as well as the biochemical results of the many emotional and mechanical environmental stresses (such as noise) that affect us. Stress, of any kind, translates into chemical messengers called *hormones*, such as cortisol or adrenalin. In other words, certain types of sensory input (such as a loud noise) can cause the nervous system, which intercepts these outside signals, to tell the adrenal glands to secrete adrenalin. The liver must process these chemicals before they can be neutralized or eliminated.

Under some circumstances, hormones can be stored by the liver for up to a year, adding fuel to emotional imbalances such as depression and anger, as well as to physical stress-related

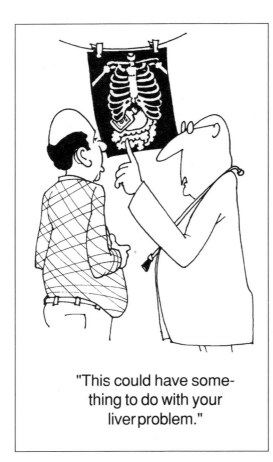

"This could have something to do with your liver problem."

imbalances such as immune system depression.

Other common liver stress factors are alcohol and recreational drugs which are prevalent in the United States. Current figures estimate 18 million alcoholics and 22 million drug abusers in this country (U.S. Congress Report, Jan. 1987; National Clearing House on Drug Addiction, 1987). Furthermore, since drugs administered for therapeutic purposes also affect the liver, 5 percent of hospital patients in the United States (1.9 million people) develop significant adverse reactions to drugs administered by doctors (U.S. Statistical Abstracts, 1984). In fact, 2 to 4 percent of all hospital admissions (760,000 to 1.5 million people) are for doctor-prescribed drug reactions. Why are there so many negative reactions to drugs? Consider that from five to ten different drugs may be administered to a hospital patient at one time. Now, as the number of drugs taken by a patient increases, the chances of unwanted cross-reactions and side effects increase exponentially.

Though many billions of dollars are spent on testing the efficacy and safety of drugs in this country, these tests are only done for drugs taken *singly*. No one knows what the effect of two or three taken together may be, much less of ten!

The Liver and Detoxification

As well as supplying and regulating the body's energy, the liver is responsible for a great deal of detoxification, which is crucial to health. As everyone knows, when garbage piles up and wastes are not removed from city streets, decay and degeneration set in—likewise with the body. When bacteria and pathogens abound in the internal environment, biochemical harmony is lost and disease sets in. Thus, since maintaining a relaxed, productive, and serene life is nearly impossible when the body is in a high state of toxicity, clean inner and outer environments are essential for health.

Now in order to understand how the liver helps to detoxify the body, we must first understand some basic chemistry. Many of the foreign and toxic chemicals that enter the body (either by descending through the food chain into the food we eat, or by direct intake of contaminants) are called *lipid-soluble*. This means they dissolve only in fatty or oily solutions, not in water. Lipid-soluble compounds have a special affinity for fat tissues and many other cells of the body which have lipid-soluble membranes, such as liver cells. These cells and tissues can store toxins for months, even years, releasing them during times of low food intake, exercise, or stress. As toxins are released, one may experience unpleasant symptoms such as tiredness, dizziness, nausea, racing pulse, etc.

It is the liver's job to transform lipid-soluble chemicals into water-soluble compounds so that they are not stored in the body but released via the kidneys and bowels instead. This transformation is carried out by a complex system of enzymes that are made in the *hepatocytes*, or liver cells.

Besides having a complex system of enzymes to remove toxic compounds from the blood, the liver also has filtering channels, called *sinusoids*, that are lined with special cells which engulf and break down foreign debris, bacteria, and toxic chemicals (this process is called *phagocytosis*). However, when the liver is burdened with high levels of toxins or pathogenic organisms (such as *Candida albicans*, a major factor in yeast infections), not all of these substances can be processed and eliminated. In fact, many will be stored in the liver, eventually causing irreparable damage.

So you can see why the liver is known in natural healing to be an important organ in maintaining clean blood, because it actually does act as a sort of blood filter. Many herbalists call certain herbs good "blood purifiers." Does this mean these herbs literally scrub the blood clean? Not really. What really happens is that the herbs stimulate increased blood flow through the liver, removing congestion. At the same time they protect and stimulate liver cells, encouraging the production of enzymes and helping to maintain a proper biochemical environment.

Of course, the liver is not the only organ involved in detoxification. Blood purification also depends upon the proper functioning of all the eliminative organs in the body. The skin, for instance, eliminates large quantities of toxins through sweating. That's why sweating and increased fluid intake can take a load off the liver, and thus help support the whole digestive process by increasing the liver's efficiency and available energy.

An Amazing Chemical Factory

The liver is really an amazing chemical factory, and some of its workings deserve further discussion.

Vitamins

Vitamins, minerals, and enzymes are vital to the body's cellular health. They are the "messengers" and "currency" that help make things happen—from the creation of new cells, to the making of sexual hormones, to the release of energy. Significantly, the liver stores vitamins and minerals for times when they would otherwise be lacking. It can store enough vitamin A to supply an adult's needs for up to four years and enough vitamin D and vitamin B12 to last for four months!

Bile

The liver also creates bile which, in some ways, acts like detergent: it helps break down fats by *emulsifying* them. Emulsification is a process that transforms large fat globules into tiny ones which are more soluble and assimilable. To help the liver with this process, a moderate walk after a meal rich in fat is desirable. This encourages the fat to move through the body and facilitates its processing.

Excessive amounts of fat and protein in the diet are difficult for the liver to break down because they make the liver work harder to produce bile and other digestive enzymes. In addition, compounds produced by the metabolic breakdown of protein, such as ammonia, can irritate or even be toxic to the liver. Thus, when the liver is not functioning properly, or if it is diseased, it is important to eat fewer foods that contain fat and protein, such as meat and dairy products. It is also good to eat more easily assimilated complex carbohydrates, such as rice or millet, because these decrease the amount of bile needed and thus take a great load off the liver. This will also help to build up and better utilize glycogen in the hepatocytes, which means the liver will have more energy to rebuild itself and establish proper harmony.

One major cause of impaired bile flow in this country is gallstones. Current medical literature states that at least 20 million people in the United States have gallstones. Bile stagnation can also result from actual cellular damage to the liver due to the negative effects of alcohol, hyperthyroidism or thyroxine supplementation, exposure to toxic drugs or other synthetic chemicals, and the use of birth control pills. When the bile is stagnant, the skin becomes sallow, yellow, or blemished. Also, important vitamins are not assimilated properly, which can impair blood clotting, vision, and the body's antioxidant system. Further damage to the body may occur when toxic compounds that are usually cycled through the bile and eliminated are held in the liver instead.

That bile is a vital bodily fluid was well understood by many ancient systems of healing. Herbs have been commonly taken throughout the world to restore proper bile flow, for when the bile is stagnant, sadness and disharmony can result. The word "melancholy," for instance, comes from the Greek *melanos* (black) and *chole* (bile)—or literally, "black bile." This condition has been called "sluggish liver" in Western medicine and "liver stagnation" in Traditional Chinese Medicine.

Enzymes
An enzyme is an agent that facilitates the transformation of

one substance into another. As we have already seen, during the detoxification process the liver makes use of various enzymes.

"toxic alkaloids in the medicinal plant comfrey are probably harmless until they travel through the liver"

Actually, these are not individual enzymes but whole enzyme systems, collectively named the Microsomal Enzyme System (MES). The MES is part of our evolutionary legacy. Its job is to process many different kinds of chemicals, as already explained. Most likely, the liver developed these enzyme systems to deactivate and facilitate the elimination of naturally occurring, endogenous (i.e., produced within the body) chemicals, such as the hormones estradiol, testosterone, bilirubin, and serotonin. The MES probably also evolved to help detoxify and eliminate many natural toxins present in the wild and in slightly spoiled foods, which were common before the advent of refrigeration.

However, the MES is a two-edged sword. On the one hand, it can transform fat-soluble toxic chemicals, such as DDT, into more water-soluble ones that are easily eliminated via the bowels and urine. But on the other hand, ironically, the MES can also transform certain recently created or even naturally occurring compounds, which are normally non-toxic, into toxic or even carcinogenic ones. For example, toxic alkaloids found in the medicinal plant comfrey are probably harmless until they travel through the liver and are transformed into highly potent compounds that can lead to liver damage. Although just how toxic these compounds are is still controversial, both researchers and herbalists are recommending caution in the use of comfrey products, especially during pregnancy. The sad truth is that our body, in all its evolutionary history, has never had to deal with the thousands of new chemicals humans are unleashing on the environment today. How these compounds interact with the myriad natural chemicals in food plants and medicinal herbs in the liver is anybody's guess.

Now the different kinds of enzyme systems in the MES have been classified into two types: Phase I and Phase II systems. Phase I systems *alter* chemical groups on the foreign substance, rendering it more water-soluble and hence disposable through the urine. Phase II systems, in contrast, generally help to *conjugate* (or bind) a compound with sulfur-containing groups, presumably to make them less toxic, or as in the case of endogenous hormones, to deactivate them.

An example of a Phase I enzyme system is the Mixed-Function Oxidases (MFO) system, part of which is the Cytochrome P-450 system. Cytochrome P-450 plays a central role in detoxifying numerous potentially hazardous compounds. It also assists the synthesis of steroid hormones and, with vitamin C, works in an important step of bile synthesis. Unfortunately for the liver, however, certain toxic chemicals disrupt the P-450 system. These include common herbicides and pesticides, as well as breakdown products from them that can linger in the environment for many years (for instance DDE, a breakdown product from DDT, is still abundant in the environment many years after DDT was banned). These can be stored in fat tissues and slowly released into the bloodstream, eventually finding their way to the liver. Because the production of synthetic pesticides exceeds 1.4 billion pounds a year in this country, it is likely that there are enough toxic substances in the environment to adversely affect our livers and lives.

"Glutathione (GSH-T) is one of the most important endogenous antioxidants in the body"

Phase II systems, for their part, include both UDP-glucuronyl transferase (GT), and glutathione-S-transferase (GSH-T). Glutathione (GSH-T) is one of the most important endogenous antioxidants and cellular protectants in the body. It can be depleted by large amounts of drugs or toxic chemicals passing through the liver, as well as by fasting or starvation. (GSH-T) is also subject to circadian rhythms, which means that its levels increase and decrease according to the body's 24-hour biological cycles. Thus there is 30 percent less GSH-T in the body in the late afternoon than late at night.

So what does all this mean for our health? Well, while natural amounts of substances such as GT and GSH-T are vital to optimal liver functioning, excessive amounts may be harmful. High GSH-T levels in the liver can cause non-toxic chemicals to be transformed into more toxic ones that damage the liver (Salbe and Bjeldanes, 1985). Thus, there must be just enough GHS-T available for important enzymatic reactions, but not so much as to cause excessive transformations. Or in other words, health depends upon biochemical *tone*. Tone means that there is just enough of a particular substance, action, or force to maintain a state of dynamic balance in the body and consequently the ability to function. The muscles are a simple example of this principle. When the arm muscles are exercised just the right amount in relation to each other, the arm can work efficiently. However, if the muscles are over- or under-stimulated, the arm becomes either too flabby or too tight to function. The Chinese call such dynamic equilibrium the balance of Yin and Yang, but many Westerners prefer the concept of tone. Everything is governed by tone—nervous activity, muscle activity, hormonal activity, and all other biochemical reactions as well. Some simple but effective ways to maintain proper tone in the GSH-T and the liver's other enzyme systems include exercise, positive attitude, visualization, polarity therapy, and various other common methods for bringing about greater health. Also, we can use herbs and diet, which we shall soon address in depth.

The Liver and Emotional Balance

In the preceding pages we have discussed a lot of technical and scientific concepts. How do these relate to the everyday lives of thinking, feeling human beings? Well, most importantly, any emotions we feel have a basis in biochemistry. When we feel angry, for instance, a complex mixture of hormones and other chemicals speed to various parts of our bodies, readying us for action. Likewise fear, jealousy, joy, sorrow, and all our other emotions have a corresponding chemical reality which can create profound changes in our bodies. And depending on the strength and duration of emotions, these changes can more or less determine one's character and outlook on life.

Thus, an important function of the liver, which is just now beginning to be understood, is its role in transforming and removing excess hormones from the blood. When the liver is diseased or is functioning poorly, its ability to do this is impaired. Emotional states that should come and go easily stay around far longer than necessary. If one's environment is full of negative emotions, or any excessive emotions, this burdens the liver.

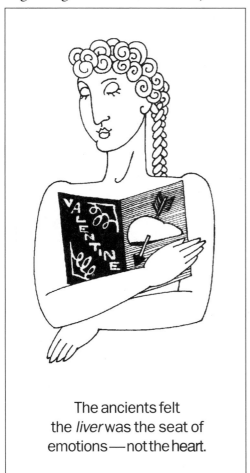

The ancients felt the *liver* was the seat of emotions — not the heart.

Take anger, for instance. In many cultures, anger is thought to reside in the liver or gallbladder (an associated organ). As detailed shortly, Traditional Chinese Medicine (TCM) holds that anger is associated with the liver and gallbladder (in a Western view we would say that the bile in the gallbladder can store the excess hormones not eliminated by a poorly functioning liver). Similarly, Ayurvedic medicine associates anger with the fire principle and the liver. Thus in both cases someone who is chronically angry would be said to have an unhealthy liver or gallbladder. The prescribed treatment would be gentle opening, cleansing, and perhaps cooling of the bile and liver, using herbs, liver flushes, and intestinal cleansing (we will discuss all of these in detail later).

The Liver and PMS

Having understood this much about the liver and the emotions, it should be easy to grasp their connection with premenstrual syndrome (PMS). Currently, PMS is being linked to excess estrogen, a steroid hormone. Again, it is the liver's job to clear away any excess estrogen circulating through the body. However, if the body produces too much estrogen, the liver may not be able to keep up with its job, resulting in PMS symptoms, such as depression, cramps, headaches, fatigue, or even more serious problems. For instance, excess estrogen has been reported to increase the risk of gallbladder disease, production of clots and inflammation in the blood vessels, high blood pressure, hyperglycemia, and breast, uterine, liver, and vaginal cancer (Physician's Desk Reference, 1983). This doesn't sound too beneficial for one's health, does it?

Natural liver therapies can help with all types of hormonal imbalances including PMS. For women who do not produce enough estrogen and consequently receive prescribed estrogen therapy (as for osteoporosis and symptoms associated with menopause), it is especially important to support the liver with natural liver therapies during times when estrogen is taken. As for those who suffer from estrogen excess leading to emotional swings, food cravings, and other undesirable symptoms, natural plant remedies can protect the body from the effects of too much estrogen blocking the binding sites estrogen normally uses to activate or modify cellular processes in estrogen-sensitive tissue, such as the lining of the uterus. In this way, some naturally occurring plant hormones, called *phytosterols*, can prevent estrogen from over-extending the scope and amount of its beneficial activities (Farnsworth, 1980).

Besides estrogen, testosterone, too, is metabolized by the liver. Testosterone normally exists in both the male and female body and is known to affect levels of aggressiveness and sexual

---

Table 3
Major Functions of the Liver

- Metabolizes proteins, fats, and carbohydrates, thus providing energy and nutrients
- Stores vitamins, minerals, and sugars
- Filters the blood and helps remove harmful chemicals and bacteria
- Creates bile, which breaks down fats
- Helps assimilate and store fat-soluble vitamins (A, E, D, K)
- Stores extra blood, which can be quickly released when needed
- Creates serum proteins, which maintain fluid balance and act as carriers
- Helps maintain electrolyte and water balance
- Creates immune substances, such as gamma globulin
- Breaks down and eliminates excess hormones

energy. Hence if the liver cannot properly eliminate excess testosterone, over-aggressiveness, extreme mood swings, and abnormal levels of sexual energy may result, as well as dysfunction of the reproductive cycle.

🍎 🍎 🍎

These then are some of the liver's major functions—vitamins, bile, enzymes, and cleansing—though it has other important functions as well (see Reynolds, 1980b for more details). Table 3 (p. 31) summarizes the liver's major functions.

The Chinese Liver System

So far we have discussed the liver as it is known to Western science. The concept of the liver in Traditional Chinese Medicine (TCM) is somewhat different and merits closer study.

According to TCM, the liver's main job is to regulate the flow of chi (*chi* means, approximately, "life energy"). Chi is responsible for all activity of the body, the blood, the chi itself, and for proper functioning of the organs. The liver moves the blood and chi smoothly in all directions throughout the body and harmonizes the functioning of the organs. Naturally, then, the liver is particularly sensitive to anything that disrupts what the Chinese so aptly call its "free and easy wanderer" movement and influence within the body. Excessive or negative emotions, especially, will disrupt this free-flowing ambience, leading to conditions of deficiency, coldness, or stagnation. The net result of any such blockage of energy in the liver is a buildup of toxins, which can cause cellular damage and poor functioning of the Microsomal Enzyme System (MES) we discussed earlier. This in turn may lead to further damage from free radicals and peroxidized lipids, which we shall address later.

As well as being susceptible to blockage or chi stagnation, the liver is also susceptible to over-stimulation. In the latter condition, the liver receives too much blood and goes into a sort of metabolic overdrive called "blazing fire" in TCM. This state can be caused by alcohol, drugs, and an excess of certain spices, such as black pepper. Blazing fire can remain localized in the liver and cause overheating, which in Western terms may lead to enzyme dysfunction and damage to the hepatocytes. Or the heat can rise up to the head, inducing headaches, facial flushing, thirst, dizziness, and ringing in the ears.

The liver has other important functions in TCM besides regulating the flow of chi in the body. First of all, it regulates digestive activity. When the liver fails in this task due to loss of biochemical harmony, its action can "invade," or negatively affect, the stomach, thus precipitating digestive problems such as abdominal pain, nausea, burping, and diarrhea.

Secondly, in TCM just as in Western medicine the liver also controls the bile. If the bile does not flow smoothly, jaundice, loss of appetite, and a bitter taste in the mouth will result. Fats will not be well tolerated or assimilated, and the fat-soluble vitamins A, E, D, and K will not be utilized well—which could lead to immune depression.

Thirdly, the liver harmonizes the emotions. According to some TCM texts, it has a "sprinkling" movement that is responsible for maintaining a relaxed and flowing inner environment and an even-tempered disposition. This works in a cyclic way: a healthy liver helps maintain an even temperament, and vice versa. However, if the cycle turns downward, a turbulent emotional climate can damage the liver, and the injured liver will further aggravate the emotional chaos.

A fourth important function of the liver, understood by TCM and Western medicine alike, is to store extra blood for use in times of need, as during physical activity. However, according to TCM, imbalances occur if the liver either does not have enough extra blood stored (resulting in dryness in the eyes), or if it loses its ability to store blood properly (resulting in excessive menstrual flow).

Lastly, it is important to note that TCM texts state that the liver also "rules" the tendons and is manifested in the nails. This can provide helpful diagnostic information. For example, if the tendons are stiff, hard, and painful, or if the nails are pale and brittle, then it could mean the liver is failing to nourish them properly.

Remember in TCM all these aspects of liver functioning are interrelated and resonant, so in reality no one aspect can be separated from the others. We only look at them separately because this helps us draw conclusions about functional dishar-mony and successful treatment.

The chart on the following page presents the major liver syndromes in TCM and their Western correlates.

ॐॐॐ

This completes the discussion of how our liver works in our behalf, but this is really only half of the whole picture. The other half is perhaps even more important—an understanding of what foods and other nutritional elements, as well as herbs that can help support and protect the liver. For basic dietary guidelines and sources of nutritional factors that can help insure liver health, see

The Liver

Therapeutic Syndrome	Western Symptoms	Principle	Correlation
stagnant or constrained liver chi	depression, anger, frustration, lumps in neck or breast, poor digestion	dredge liver, promote bile flow	congested liver, blood flow constrained
deficient liver yin/uprising liver yang	dizziness, blurry vision or night blind-ness, flushed face	tonify the yin, pacify the liver, subdue the yang	deficient in enzymes and other substances besides blood and energy
blazing liver fire	hypertension, migraine	clear liver, purge fire	excess sympathetic nervous stimula-tion, liver over-worked
liver blood deficiency/ poor blood storage	weakness of tendons or ligaments, poor digestion	tonify blood, nurture liver	liver blood supply constrained, anemia, protein deficiency
liver wind moving	body rigidity, extreme dizziness, severe pain	pacify liver, extinguish wind	bile blockage, nerve disorders, ten-sion in muscles

the Diet and Food Chapter, p. 36. For herbs and herbal programs, both western and Chinese, that can help protect and rebuild liver function, see the Herbal Therapy Chapter, p. 106.

Chapter 3

Diet and Food Therapy
For the Liver and Digestion

General Dietary Guidelines

When one considers the entire evolution of humankind, our modern dietary excursion into the world of processed foods is of very recent history. Given that the human race has perhaps evolved over half a million years eating foods such as seeds, grains, fruits, and wild greens, 50 or 100 years is not nearly enough time for our biochemistry to adjust to the bland, sugary, high-fat diet that is predominantly consumed today. The question we must pose ourselves, then, is what exactly constitutes a balanced diet in the modern world?

Diet is a confusing topic because there seem to be so many different kinds of diets out there. However, when you take away the fads and the lose-weight-quickly shams, the remaining proponents all agree on one thing: **it is best to eat food in its most whole, unprocessed state.** The more refined a food is, the less vital energy it has. Beyond that, there seem to be two major camps in diet philosophy: the raw-fooders and the macrobiotic fans. Raw-food enthusiasts say that when food is cooked it loses vital energy and enzymes and is much more likely to ferment or decompose in the intestines, leading to a toxic state of the body. Macrobiotic proponents say that warming or cooking food makes it easier to digest, especially for those with weakened digestion.

They believe that raw food, especially, may "cool" the digestion so much that it becomes dysfunctional.

Which way is right? The Japanese have lived by macrobiotic-style dietary guidelines for centuries—it is their traditional way of eating. And before Western processed foods started becoming popular in Japan, the Japanese were a very healthy people. On the other hand, one of the leading proponents of the raw-food diet, Norman Walker, was recently reported to have died at the age of 115. Of course, it must be mentioned that he lived in Arizona, a hot and dry climate where raw foods make a suitable diet. Nonetheless, he must have been doing something right!

My own feeling is that elements from both diets are worth considering. Depending on one's type of work, emotional makeup, body constitution, the climate one lives in, and the season, one may need raw foods at times, and lightly steamed vegetables and warmed grains and legumes at other times. I practiced a nearly raw-food diet for several years and found it to be satisfactory for that time. I had tremendous energy and was rarely sick. I did find, though, that sometimes I had trouble being as steady in my work as I would have liked to be—but that may have been a reflection of who I was at the time. During the last eight years, I have been eating more whole grains and other starches, tofu, tempeh, and also raw salads. I have been healthy—provided I don't try to work too hard or do excessive mental work, which can be extremely ruinous to the health.

All in all, then, I would say that systems are useful as guidelines to follow, but it is important to remember that each of us is so unique that eventually, for our own optimum health, we must find our own personal system. Nevertheless, after many years of study and experimentation, I have developed a few simple, general rules about diet that should apply to most people.

1. **Never worry about what we eat**. We may consistently and gently remind ourselves about habits we know are bad, but we should not worry. In the moment we are eating, be it a greasy burger or the finest organic brown rice, we should always relax and enjoy what we eat.

2. **Do not overeat**. Neither should we eat too late at night, or in the morning before doing some exercise.

3. **Eat high-quality, whole, unprocessed food.** So much of our food is processed, allowing it to remain on the shelf for months, as well as increasing the profit margins for the manufacturer. To really bring this point into focus, try walking through a modern "convenience" store and take a close look at the food products that are displayed. If one is interested in the energetically highest food, the food that creates the highest health, there is really nothing there to eat!

4. **Choose food suitable to our constitution, work, and climate.** After 22 years as a strict vegetarian, recently I began to develop signs of deficiency, such as weak lower back and knees. In Traditional Chinese Medicine (TCM), these are symptoms of "kidney Qi" deficiency. Since I am a student and practitioner of TCM, I decided to follow the guidelines of this ancient system of medicine by adding some fish to my diet 2 or 3 times a week. This was not easy for me to do after so many years of not eating any kind of meat, but balancing the many good reasons for not eating animals was my desire to avoid being too rigid. It is important to experiment in one's life. Conditions and needs are never static, and true health is found through the ability to change our ideas with changing environmental and internal conditions. I will discuss several important issues regarding

vegetarianism in paragraph 8. I can say that moderate amounts of fish have made a positive difference in my health. Since humans are probably omnivorous by nature, small amounts of meat may be helpful as medicine for some people. However, most people would benefit from less meat in their diet and even periods of abstinence.

5. **Eat about a 60-70% cooked, high-carbohydrate diet**. Emphasize a variety of organic whole grains, legumes, and vegetables, and de-emphasize flour products like breads and muffins.

6. **Keep raw fruit (including fruit juices) to a minimum.** Unless we live in a hot climate, it is best to eat fruit moderately during the summer and only sparingly during the winter, unless we are consciously following a cleansing diet for a time. Young people, who are usually hotter by nature, also tend to do well on fresh fruits. We may eat more raw vegetables and salads than fruit in all seasons, but be aware that raw foods, and especially raw fruits, are cooling, moisturizing, and induce elimination. This is fine if we have a hot, dry constitution and a buildup of excessive fat or toxic wastes, or if we live in a hot, dry climate. However, if we have a cold, moist, and deficient condition, eating large amounts of raw foods can be harmful. In this case, eat mostly cooked grains, vegetables and legumes, and some fish or meat, where indicated.

7. **Remain open to change, experimentation, and growth.** Remember there is no "absolutely" correct dietary system. This point is highlighted in the next and last guideline, below.

8. **Vegetarianism or not?** After having practiced strict vegetarianism for over 22 years myself, and having spoken with many other vegetarians, I feel qualified to speak from experience

on the topic of vegetarianism. However, because it is such a personal matter, the final decision of whether or not to eat animal flesh must, of course, rest with each individual.

As I see it, the main issues regarding vegetarianism fall into four general areas: spiritual and ethical issues; environmental concerns; and physical health matters.

Spiritual and Ethical Issues

The spiritual teachers I have admired the most have all emphasized the need for following a vegetarian diet. The reasons given are respect for life, non-violence, and the avoidance of karmic debt. Although meat-eaters have often told me that plants can feel, too, and don't like to be killed for food, I think there is much more violence involved in killing an animal than in plucking the leaves or fruit from a plant or tree, or even pulling up a whole carrot or beet. This difference of degree is quickly evident if you take a short walk through a slaughterhouse and listen to the animals' shrieks of terror and death-cries. When I hear this, I feel in my soul that such unrestrained killing incurs karmic debt. Also, my teachers have told me that killing animals, because they embody all the elements (i.e., fire, air, water, earth, ether), involves more karmic debt than killing plants, which contain only the air, water, and earth elements. The only spiritually and ethically conscious way of killing animals, as I see it, is to do so as the Native Americans did, with prayers and reverence, giving thanks for the gift of the animal's life, and acknowledging that one day, we will serve as food for the plants, trees, and ultimately other animals.

Environmental Considerations

This is one area where vegetarianism wins out hands down. There is no question that agriculture is a more land-efficient way of sustaining people than raising livestock. Indeed, this is the common argument given to explain why vegetarianism is so widespread in India. In the United States, 64% of cropland is used to feed livestock, while only 2% is needed to produce our massive quantities of fruits and vegetables. Further, one-half of all water used is for livestock. And then there is the daily destruction of the tropical rainforests, which can be more than partially blamed on the meat-eating habits in the Standard American Diet (SAD). Given the starving millions in the world today, as well as what future generations must face in light of the population explosion, can we really make meat a daily choice? With more people on the planet, we need to eat in a more energy-efficient way.

Also, being a botanist myself, it has been particularly heart-wrenching to witness the widespread destruction of natural habitats all over the U.S. caused by grazing cows. This destruction occurs even in national parks and forests, which one might consider protected. I have been in the high Sierras and seen pristine mountain wildflower meadows turned into quagmires of muddy hoof-holes. I have seen the beautiful California woodlands all over the state being overgrazed, with the result that native wildflowers have been replaced by weedy mono-cultures of wild oats, thistles, and black mustard. Many of these habitats may be lost forever.

If people got into the habit of eating less red meat and more grains, legumes, and vegetables, we could preserve thousands of acres of natural habitat—habitat which is home not only for many wildflowers, but also for numerous animal and bird species as well.

Physical Health Matters

The physical health aspects of meat-eating are the least clear of the issues in my experience. On one hand, there is no doubt that most people eat too much meat—especially red meat, which has been shown to lead to increased risk of bowel cancer and cardio-vascular disease. However, on the other hand, is there ever a case where a person is not getting enough meat? Strict vegetarians say no, but in some traditional systems of healing, especially Tradi-tional Chinese Medicine (TCM) and Ayurveda, it is thought that people who are very weak or deficient may benefit from meat. In this context, the meat is taken in small amounts and is considered more like a medicine than a staple. Over the years, I have met people who have been vegetarians for years, but who eventually became weak and deficient and suffered diseases such as chronic fatigue syndrome, general immune weakness, and other health problems. I have also seen their conditions improve when they reintroduced small amounts of meat into their diets.

In fact, I myself have had this experience. As mentioned above, after many years as a vegetarian, I developed symptoms of deficiency, such as weak knees and lower back, tiredness, and feelings of spaciness. After eating fish once or twice a week for several months, I felt stronger and more substantial. In the last 6 months before I started eating fish, I was only able to swim about half a mile before feeling weak and dizzy. After I had eaten fish for a month, I could swim for a mile or more easily, with no feelings of weakness. Of course, I am the first to admit that this is by no means a controlled experiment. There may have been

The Safety of Meat

When eating meat, it is important to identify "safe meat." Keep in mind that most commercial meats, such as hatchery-raised salmon, as well as beef, chicken, and turkey, are often raised with the use of steroids, antibiotics, and other synthetic chemicals. Because of this, I recommend considering avoidance of these. For those who eat red meat, look for custom-raised meat from farms or ranches that use organic methods. Organically-raised chickens and turkeys are also available.

Salmon, though a very nourishing fish, is often hatchery grown, likely with the use of synthetic chemicals. Some wild races of salmon are nearing extinction. Because of these important reasons, I have stopped eating salmon, and now eat only deep sea fish such as red snapper or halibut. Fish that are higher on the food chain, such as shark or swordfish, may have more concentrated levels of environmental pollutants than smaller fish. Finally, it is important to look at which species have been under strong commercial pressure. Tuna, for instance, is becoming rare.

Because animals eat plants, they generally concentrate more environmental toxins, such as heavy metals, in their tissues. This may become an increasing concern over the next number of years, if more and more industrial and public waste is dumped without regard for the consequences. It is good to keep in mind that we can make a difference—reversing this trend by becoming environmental activists. We can write our representatives and demand that they support legislation that requires putting our environment first before all other concerns. If not, what will be left for our children?

other factors to consider, e.g., perhaps I was resting more and thinking less. Who is to say? But my intuition (which I trust) tells me that the meat protein did give me more strength. On the other hand, there are those people who never seem to have problems with a vegetarian diet. In any case, I do believe that practicing long-term vegetarianism requires great care and attention. It requires eating a varied and balanced diet of high-quality foods, as well as resting and going inward and not over-extending oneself. This is often difficult in our fast-paced modern lifestyle, given work, family, and other obligations. In conclusion, I will say that I have no idea how long I will continue to eat fish, but I believe that I will know when to eat it and when not to, provided I listen closely to what my body is telling me. At first, eight months ago, I ate fish 2-3 times weekly, but now I seem to require it only once every week or 10 days.

I feel there is one question we must always ask ourselves when we decide to eat meat. Do I really need this for my health and well-being? If the meat is for pleasure or is eaten out of habit or an unhealthy craving, it may be best to reexamine one's motives and choose to eat vegetables, grains, and legumes instead.

Food Energetics: Flavor Therapy

In the West we have become accustomed to hearing about the need to represent all the basic food groups in our diet, i.e., meat, starch, dairy products, vegetables, and fruits. Traditional Chinese Medicine, however, has a different concept of what a balanced diet is. In TCM, one speaks of the need to include all the basic *flavor* groups in the diet. The following chart shows the basic flavors and their corresponding organs.

The Organs and Their Associated Tastes

Taste	Organ	Effects
Sweet	Spleen	enhances immunity, energy
Sour	Liver	detoxifies
Bitter	Heart	protects, activates assimilation
Acrid (spicy)	Lungs	clears, opens, warms
Salty	Kidneys	regulates water, electrolyte, and nerve balance

Thus, in TCM, the liver's curative flavor is *sour*, which cools and cleanses (lemon juice and schisandra berries are examples of sour tastes). For thousands of years the Chinese have based curative dietary and herbal combinations upon these flavor groups. This actually makes good scientific sense since flavors are powerful activators of the digestive tract and other organ systems, and throughout history the human body has always associated the flavors of foods with the release of enzymes to break down and assimilate specific nutrients. Taste has always been the first clue as to which of the many digestive enzymes the body needs to produce in order to digest a particular kind of food.

Today, however, flavors no longer provide this vital link to digestion because we have altered our food chemistry so extensively. Even when we do eat vegetables in their whole state, we mainly buy them from a supermarket spread of tasteless genetic creations bred for looks and texture rather than for character of flavor. One need only think of the difference between the bitter, salty, rich flavor of dandelion greens, as opposed to watery and tasteless iceberg lettuce. Red delicious apples are quite flavorless when compared to a wild apple, or even a good pippin.

So how can we enjoyably add more therapeutic tastes to our diet? Besides herbal remedies, each of which has a unique flavor or blend of flavors, I have found that condiments offer the best opportunity for "taste enhancement." Whether I am at home or on the road talking about herbs and health, I usually have some kind of condiment at hand to add to the foods I eat. Traditional cultures know the value of all the tastes in a meal, and often one can find many interesting side-dishes, relishes, and other condiments in ethnic restaurants. Unfortunately, though, modern American culture seems to have lost this "spice of life."

The dramatic difference between our own national cuisine and that of many other traditional cultures was brought home to me recently. An old friend of the family wanted to meet me in town for lunch and was adamant that we meet in one of those plastic chain restaurants I like to stay out of. So, as I sat there at the table, I noticed that the only condiments on the table were salt and pepper. Now this scene would not have surprised me when I was growing up—it is a very normal one in most restaurants. But today, after having had a large tray of interesting and flavorful condiments on my own table for so many years, I couldn't help but notice the difference.

The following chart presents the five flavors and some of the readily available condiments and spices that have them. Bon appétit!

Condiments and Spices for Good Digestion

<u>Taste</u>	<u>Condiment</u>
Bitter	bitter melon, lemon pickle, fresh parsley, parsley flakes, wild greens powder*
Sour	pickled ginger, sauerkraut, pepperoncini peppers, kim-chi, lemon, vinegar
Salty	kelp, nori, wakame, and other seaweeds, parsley, celery, gamasio, umeboshi plum paste
Spicy	peppers, stone-ground mustard, pickled ginger, hot sauces, salsa
Sweet	maple syrup, brown rice syrup, barley malt, honey, stevia herb, unrefined cane sugar, date sugar

*See the recipe for wild greens powder on p. 50. Also, see Chapter 5, "Herbal Therapy," for a discussion of bitter herbs and their many benefits, pages 115-122.

Superfoods: Wild Greens for the Picking

Wild greens—nature's superfoods—are probably the most overlooked dietary resource in this country. Wild greens are easy to grow. Just collect wild plant seeds, such as mallow, yellow dock, sheep sorrel, plantain, sow thistle, and dandelion, and let them go in your yard or garden. They ask for little in the way of upkeep and space and will give bountifully in return. Or, if you prefer, just gather the wild greens that grow naturally in your yard, vacant lot, field, or meadow near your home (watch for chemical sprays, though, and pick at least 100 feet from a main road.) These "pot herbs," as they are called, are eagerly sought and used on a daily basis in many countries around the world. I have seen people pick wild greens in Asia, Greece, England, Germany, and other parts of Europe. Rarely or never do I see people making use of even the most delectable and sweet wild greens in the United States—proving, again, that we have lost a lot of common sense in dietary matters. The "food-consumer culture" created by the food-processing giants in this country has instilled the idea that if food doesn't come from a store such as Safeway (the name itself is proof), it isn't fit or safe to eat.

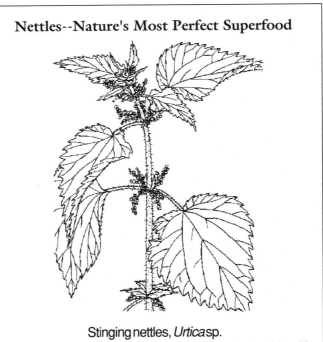

Nettles--Nature's Most Perfect Superfood

Stinging nettles, *Urtica* sp.
Nettles can be steamed and eaten as a green vegetable with lemon juice, seaweed, or other condiments or dried and powdered in the Supergreens blend. Nettles contain extraordinarily high amounts of minerals, vitamins and chlorophyll, and 3.5% high-quality protein.

Table 4
Properties and Nutritional Value of Wild Greens
(mg/100 gm unless otherwise stated)

Plant	Tastes	Iron	Magnesium	Calcium	Vitamin A
Dandelion greens	bitter	4 mg	36 mg	187 mg	14000 IU
Dock greens	sour, bitter	2 mg	—	66 mg	12900 IU
Lamb's quarters	salty, sour	1 mg	—	309 mg	11600 IU
Purslane	sour, demulcent	4 mg	—	79 mg	750 IU
Nettles	salty	9 mg	—	212 mg	—
Mallow	demulcent	19 mg	—	312 mg	2.53 mg
Chickweed	sweet	3 mg	30 mg	20 mg	1000 IU
Amaranth (pigweed)	salty, bitter	6 mg		313 mg	1599 IU
Kelp	salty, sweet	100 mg	760 mg	1093 mg	2 IU
Watercress	salty, spicy	2 mg	20 mg	151 mg	4900 IU

While many wild greens are mildly bitter (helping to activate digestion), others, such as miner's lettuce, lamb's quarters, and chickweed, are every bit as sweet and juicy as the finest cultivated lettuce, and much more flavorful and nutritious!

The nutritional value of wild greens far surpasses that of their domestic cousins. Dandelion greens, for instance, have a whopping 14,000 IU of vitamin A (for 100 grams of edible leaves) compared to 330 IU for iceberg lettuce—not really in the same league! Since the daily requirement set for vitamin A is 5,000 IU, only 1 1/4 ounces of steamed dandelion greens would be sufficient for a day's supply. Compare that with 3 1/3 pounds of iceberg lettuce to provide the same amount! Table 4 lists the nutrient values of various types of wild greens.

Wild Greens Powder

Pick only undamaged, green, healthy leaves of several species of the following wild greens. Make up your own blend based on the greens available in your area.

Yellow dock (*Rumex crispus*)
Mallow (*Malva* sp.)
Dandelion (*Taraxacum officinale*)
Chicory (*Cichorium intybus*)
Plantain (*Plantago* sp.)
Nettles (*Urtica* sp.)

Dry these leaves thoroughly using moderate heat, then powder them well and store the powder in amber glass jars. To use, place some of the powder in a shaker-top jar and sprinkle on food.

Note: when picking nettles, use gloves to avoid being stung. After drying, the sting is deactivated.

Fats and Oils

One of the greatest potential dangers in the modern diet is the kinds and quantities of fats and oils we consume. This is particularly pertinent to the liver, as it is a major site where fats and oils accumulate and are processed. Recently we have embraced the use of more unsaturated fats in our diets because of the bad press saturated fats have received concerning their role in heart disease, a leading cause of death in industrial countries. Manufacturers are now touting foods containing unsaturated oils as being healthy and natural. The sad truth, though, is that in trading saturated fats for unsaturated oils, we may only be trading heart disease for cancer, premature aging, excessive skin wrinkles, and liver damage.

How so? Well, it relates to how oxygen affects fats and oils in the body. Oxygen is the key element in the basic metabolic process of *oxidation*, that is, burning up and breaking down nutrients and other molecules—or what we more commonly call metabolism. Many of the body's chemical reactions depend upon oxygen as a sort of catalytic fuel. However, because oxygen is a very reactive element, it doesn't always stick to only helpful biochemical reactions; it can also create harmful reactions by oxidizing various susceptible substances. Unsaturated oils are highly prone to such dangerous oxidation due to their double bonds that link carbon atoms together), which are easily attacked by oxygen.

Oil that has been oxidized becomes rancid. It should never be eaten because doing so can lead to the creation of *free radicals* in the body. Free radicals are molecules that are highly reactive to certain parts of healthy cells, such as cell-wall components and

Saturated vs. Unsaturated Oils

Both animal and vegetable oils and fats are made up of molecules called fatty acids, of which there are three main kinds—saturated, unsaturated, and monosaturated fatty acids. Saturated fatty acids have more hydrogen atoms and less carbon-carbon double bonds than unsaturated fatty acids. Saturated fatty acids are usually solid at room temperature, like lard. Unsaturated fatty acids have less hydrogen atoms and more carbon-carbon double bonds. They are often liquid at room temperature, like soy oil. Monosaturated fatty acids have characteristics of both types and may be liquid at room temperature and solid when refrigerated, like olive oil, which contains mostly unsaturated and monosaturated fatty acids. Although there is still much to learn about the way the body responds to a constant diet of certain kinds of fats, we do have enough information to make a few clear statements about fats in the diet. Recent research strongly supports the idea that fresh, cold-processed oils that contain mostly unsaturated or monosaturated fatty acids are far preferable to oils that are refined and heated, or made up of mostly saturated fatty acids (like animal fat).

even DNA. It is thought by modern medical researchers that free radicals "attack" the body's cells and lead to widespread tissue damage (such as in the liver) and acceleration of the aging process. In fact, there is a free radical theory of aging, first scoffed at by researchers, that is now widely accepted. This theory holds that many signs of aging, such as loss of flexibility and function in the joints, skin, and even internal organs (especially the liver), are promoted by free radicals.

Now about 17 percent of our total oxygen consumption turns into free radicals (Levine & Kidd, 1985) that can damage lipids and other cellular molecules. Most oxygen-consuming organisms have evolved defense systems to keep such free-radical damage to tolerable levels (Quintahilha, 1985). In human beings, these natural defense mechanisms include enzyme systems, such as the glutathione (GSH-T) peroxidase system we discussed earlier; naturally occurring antioxidants such as vitamin C, A, and especially E; and DNA repair mechanisms. Nonetheless, these natural defense mechanisms did not evolve with the modern diet in mind, and they may be supplemented with healing plants that provide many of the essential elements needed to sustain our natural defense systems.

Free radicals are increasingly coming to be recognized as a serious health risk. Most of the foods found on grocery store shelves, such as chips, crackers, cookies, and others, are absolutely pernicious. The process of heating and exposing to air the many unsaturated oils these foods contain has rendered them a major source of potentially dangerous free radicals. A recent Japanese study notes that liver damage due to oxidized oils in food now has to be regarded as a serious problem for human health (Kiso, 1987). The irony of the situation, however, is that highly unsaturated, essential fatty acids, such as linoleic acid, are important for human health. I know this sounds like a double-bind—we need unsaturated oils, but they can harm us—yet everything should run smoothly if we follow nature's rules and ingest only whole, natural, and preferably unheated oils in moderate quantities. We should also provide ourselves with ample free radical protectors, or antioxidants.

Here are some general recommendations regarding oils and fats:

• **Olive oil** (extra virgin) is the most natural to our bodies, is resistant to oxidation, and contains a good balance of saturated, monosaturated, and unsaturated fatty acids.

• **Flax seed (linseed) oil** provides a rich source of essential fatty, linoleic, and linolenic acids.

• **Avoid margarine**, which contains oils that have been heated and pressurized to change their molecular structure—a biochemical nightmare for the body, especially for the liver. (Crisco is unmentionable).

• Lightly salted **raw butter** is superior to margarine. Where no refrigeration is available, **ghee** (clarified butter) can be used, because it won't rot (this is why it is used in India).

• **Unsaturated oils** (such as sunflower and safflower) should be **tasted for rancidity** (a sharp, biting taste). If they are fresh to begin with, they should be stored in the refrigerator once opened.

• As much as possible, obtain essential fatty acids and other oils the body needs from **whole nuts and seeds**, preferably raw and organically grown.

Raw nuts and seeds are the best source of high-quality, essential fatty acids and have low amounts of saturated oils. The tables on the next page give the relative amounts (in grams) of saturated and unsaturated fatty acids in common nuts and seeds, and the breakdown of the saturated and unsaturated fatty acid content of several common oils.

Table 5
Fatty Acid Composition(%)
of Some Common Fats and Oils
(Sources: Erasmus, 1986; Ensminger, 1983)

Source	% Total Saturated Fatty acids	% Oleic Acid	% Total Unsaturated Fatty acids
Butter (81% fat)	62%	25%	4%
Corn oil	17%	24%	59%
Cottonseed oil	26%	18%	52%
Lard	40%	41%	15%
Linseed oil (flax)	9%	19%	72%
Olive oil	16%	76%	8%
Palm kernel	85%	13%	2%
Peanut oil	18%	47%	29%
Rape seed oil	7%	50%	37%
Salmon (7.4% fat)	18%	18%	39%
Sesame oil	13%	42%	45%
Soybean oil	15%	26%	59%

Table 6
Fatty Acid Content of Common Nuts and Seeds
(gms/100 gms)
(Ensminger, et al., 1983)

FOOD	Total Fat	Saturated Fat	Oleic	Total Unsaturated Fat
Almonds	54.2	8%	67%	19%
Brazilnuts	66.9	26%	33%	38%
Cashew nuts	45.7	20%	57%	17%
Filberts	62.4	7%	80%	11%
Peanuts	48.7	17%	48%	24%
Sunflower	47.3	13%	19%	64%
Walnuts, English	64.0	11%	15%	6

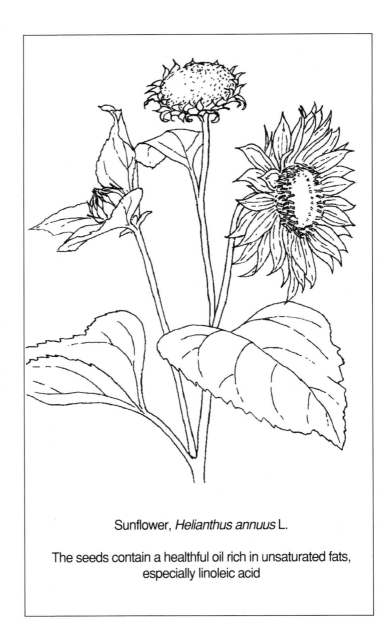

Sunflower, *Helianthus annuus* L.

The seeds contain a healthful oil rich in unsaturated fats,
especially linoleic acid

Natural Liver Therapy with Nutrition

Several kinds of foods, herbs, and other naturally occurring substances can protect and fortify the liver. These fall into five classes:

1. Antioxidants (protect cells and tissues in the liver)
2. Membrane stabilizing compounds (protect liver cells)
3. Choleretics (promote bile; help detoxify the liver)
4. Substances that prevent depletion of certain vital sulfur compounds
5. Substances that stimulate or reduce the activity of some of the liver enzyme systems

Table 7 on the following page presents one important class of liver protectors—antioxidants—and indicates nutrient sources for them. Table 8 summarizes basic dietary guidelines for maintaining liver enzymes, as discussed in The Liver chapter (Chapter 2), and specifies nutrient and whole food sources for liver builders, cleansers, and protectors. Finally, on p. 59 is a summary of basic dietary guidelines for optimum liver health.

Table 7
Sources of Liver-Protecting Substances

Antioxidants

VITAMINS
vitamin C
vitamin E
vitamin A

MINERALS
zinc
selenium

AMINO ACIDS
methionine
glutathione
cysteine

Antioxidants

FLAVONOIDS
catechin
quercetin
rutin
kaempferol
luteolin

Table 8
Natural Sources of Liver Builders, Cleansers, and Protectors

FOODS

Cleansers:
  juicy fruits (apples, vinegar)
  raw juices, vegetables

Builders:
  seeds, nuts (almonds)
  iron-rich, B-vitamin rich foods

Protectors:
  cole crops (cabbage, broccoli)

Enzyme Builders:
  cole crops
  green vegetables

Antioxidants:
  whole seeds (vit. E)
  fruit (vit. C)
  greens, red peppers (A)
  sprouts
  spirulina
  carrot juice

Table 9
Basic Dietary Guidelines For Liver Health

• **Protein**: too little or too much can disrupt liver enzymes. About 35 to 60 grams/day is optimal.

Most people in industrialized countries eat far too much protein. This places a strain on the kidneys, liver, and bowels. When bacteria in the large intestine act on protein residues, toxins are produced that may be absorbed into the bloodstream. Mother's milk is less than 2% protein, and babies require proportionally more protein than adults, because they are growing rapidly. This translates into about 30 or 40 grams/day for an adult, which is supported by looking at traditional diets around the world. Many cultures do fine on 40 grams per day. Also, vegetable protein will cause less pathogenic bacteria to grow in the intestine than meat protein, resulting in less potential for toxemia.

• **Sulfur-containing foods**: potent enzyme-builders, such as cabbage, brussel sprouts, broccoli, nuts, and seeds are all good. Take at least one serving a day of these foods—especially of vegetables from the mustard family, which provide excellent enzyme support for the liver.

• **Fats:** these are hard for the liver to process, yet provide a good energy source. A small amount of unsaturated fat is essential to health, but too much will oxidize easily, creating potentially harmful products (see section on Fats and Oils).

• **Protectors**: vitamins, minerals, herbs, amino acids, and flavonoids should be present in ample amounts. See the Natural Liver Therapy chart on p. 59. Live vegetable juices, such as carrot, beet, celery, or parsley juice, or a complete nutritional system supplement, are recommended.

• **Refined sugars**: glucose can lower enzyme activity. Humans naturally crave sweets, but when they are eaten in the highly refined form that most processed foods contain, the effectiveness of liver enzymes can be lowered. Sweet foods can be a healthful addition to the diet if they contain predominantly complex and unrefined sugars, such as those found in all fruits, vegetables, whole grains, and in barley malt and rice syrup. For a sweeter treat, use more concentrated sugars such as dates, dried fruit, pure unrefined cane sugar, and honey in moderation.

• **Phosphatidyl choline**: a constituent of lecithin that can improve the health of the microsomal membrane where enzymes are produced. Soybean products are a good source for this substance, as is phosphatidyl choline-rich lecithin, which is commercially available.

Chapter 4

Probiotics:
Beneficial Microorganisms

The Human Body as an Ecosystem

The human body is a walking ecosystem. Although we do not usually think of ourselves in this way, the fact is that we are "home" to trillions of microorganisms that live on and inside us. We are actually made up of 90% bacteria cells (100 trillion) and only 10% animal cells (10 trillion). Every person harbors more microorganisms in his or her gastrointestinal tract than there are people in the world. The gums, teeth, hair, and skin are also richly populated with many types of microorganisms.

Although some of the microorganisms inside us may be harmful, the vast majority are not. In fact, they are necessary for good health. Human beings have evolved with these microorganisms and have developed a symbiotic relationship with them. For instance, beneficial bacteria in the intestines help digest foods, create vitamins (such as B-12 and K), and inhibit the growth of disease-promoting pathogenic bacteria. Without these beneficial, or *probiotic* microorganisms, we could not survive.

Throughout history many peoples have traditionally eaten certain cultured and fermented foods that are rich in beneficial microorganisms and can increase digestive strength and general health. For instance, fermentation with lactic-acid forming bacteria, such as *Lactobacillus acidophilus,* has long been used to make cultured foods like yogurt and sauerkraut. In ancient times this process was inadvertently initiated in milk and vegetables using the organisms naturally present in the raw food, the air, or on utensils. Today genetically-selected starter cultures are used commercially, and the industry for foods and supplements that contain probiotic organisms is rapidly growing. Many scientific studies over the last 50 years have shown that probiotic organisms improve the nutritional quality of foods and can produce antibiotics, anticarcinogens, anticholesteremic substances, and substances that break down and recycle toxins (Shahani, 1983).

I will give recipes for yogurt and sauerkraut and specific recommendations for taking probiotic supplements later in this chapter. For the moment, though, let's take a closer look at what probiotic microorganisms are and what they do in the body and at the history of scientific research into this fascinating subject.

The Intestinal Microflora (IM)

In keeping with the analogy of the body as an ecosystem in itself, the rich supply of microorganisms in the intestines has been given a special name: the *intestinal microflora*, or IM as I call it for short. The IM is an amazingly complex mixture, containing an estimated 400-500 different species of bacteria (at least 17 families and 50 different genera of bacteria). Among these many species, there may be dozens—or even hundreds—of different genetic variants or biotypes. All areas of the gastrointestinal tract contain these bacteria, but the colon is by far the most heavily populated. The upper small intestine is mostly sterile, but the lower small intestine and stomach have limited numbers of various species of microorganisms, depending on conditions there. The mouth and vagina also harbor a rich microflora, which probably plays a role in the health of these areas of the body, too.

Why are there so many different species and biotypes of microorganisms in the intestines? Well, if you think of the IM

"The Intestinal Microflora is a swarming, evolving world of bacteria."

---

as a very basic physical link between our bodies and the external environment, it begins to make sense. One benefit of the complexity of the IM is to allow us to adapt to the great diversity of environments we may come into contact with. Studies show that the predominant species or biotypes of bacteria in the IM are constantly changing (Gustafsson, 1983). The IM is a swarming, evolving world of bacteria that is continually responding to changes in diet, climate, microorganisms in the environment, and other factors that have yet to be determined. Thus, if we are forced through necessity to subsist on a certain kind of food that we cannot digest very well, then the make-up of the microflora has the ability to change so that it can produce the enzymes needed to help us extract the nutrients we need from that food.

For example, most people in the United States would not do well eating large quantities of lichens. However, the Laplanders from Scandinavia eat certain lichens and gain nourishment from them—thanks to adaptations in their IM systems. Similarly, if you eat a great deal of meat, or if you eat a high-cellulose diet, your IM will adapt accordingly. So you can see that the IM might be considered a very important homeostatic mechanism in the body, helping us to survive and even thrive in varying environmental conditions. (This adaptive power of the IM has its limits, nonetheless, as we shall see later, when we discuss antibiotics.)

The IM is so vital to the human organism that Csaky went so far as to call it a separate "organ" in the body (Drasar & Hill, 1974). This designation may be extreme, but it is not without reason. The IM actually does perform some of the same functions as certain conventional organs. Like the liver, the IM breaks down complex molecules and manufactures chemicals.

Lactic Acid

Lactic acid is a simple organic acid that is found in sour milk and is a byproduct of the bacterial fermentation of many starches. It inhibits pathogenic organisms and may help remove toxins from the bowel, including some fat-soluble toxins and heavy metals. Lactic acid is largely responsible for the food-preserving qualities of fermentation (as in sauerkraut). Many probiotic microorganisms produce lactic acid to a greater or lesser extent.

However, the IM also has certain unique capabilities, such as the ability to quickly change with varying environmental and metabolic conditions. The IM can grow and regenerate much faster than the liver, and it can also secrete a much wider range of compounds than liver cells can (Drasar, 1974). In short, then, the IM is a living, adapting organ of amazing power and capacity. In this time of immense and rapid planetary changes, perhaps our need for a healthy IM is greater than ever.

Scientific Research on the Intestinal Microflora

History

The importance of the IM for human health was first brought to light by the Russian scientist Élie Metchnikoff, around the turn of the century. After years of research work with microbes, Metchnikoff became convinced that most of the degenerative diseases and aging processes that take place in humans result from toxic compounds produced by putrefactive bacteria. Interestingly, though, Metchnikoff also became convinced that certain bacteria in the body are beneficial in that they help eliminate putrefactive bacteria, and thus they may actually slow down the aging process. Metchnikoff decided that the most important of these beneficial microorganisms is *Lactobacillus bulgaricus*, a bacteria that occurs naturally in the intestines and promotes the formation of lactic acid. Metchnikoff arrived at this conclusion by studying ethnic groups, such as the Bulgarians, that have had a long history of good health. He noticed that many of these peoples have used fermented or cultured foods (like yogurt and sauerkraut), and he thus inferred that these foods may have a great potential for maintaining health. Metchnikoff also wondered whether the lactic-acid forming bacteria used to make these preserved foods might also be used to preserve human tissues from putrefaction.

In 1921, Rettger and Cheplin of Yale University conducted research on the intestinal microflora and fermented dairy foods. They suggested that *L. acidophilus* is the active organism that makes soured milk products a healthy addition to the diet, not *L.*

bulgaricus as Metchnikoff had proposed. Since then, research on the IM has continued, and various products for bolstering the IM have been made commercially available to the public. Today, interest in the IM has reached a new peak. Science still has much more to learn about the factors that affect the IM and about how exactly IM disorders cause and/or interact with various types of illnesses. Hopefully future studies will answer these questions. In the meantime, following is a review of what research has shown so far about probiotics.

Beneficial Activities of Probiotic Organisms

There are two ways to approach the subject of the probiotic organisms that constitute the IM. One way is to look at the positive roles that these organisms play in the body. The other is to study factors that negatively affect or harm them. To start on a positive note, let's look first at the benefits of having abundant probiotic organisms in the body.

Below I have gathered information on eleven main points of interest. These are the major benefits of adding probiotic organisms to the diet, whether in a pure form, such as with *L. acidophilus* supplements, or in the form of traditional fermented and cultured foods. Please note that some of these benefits have been definitively established, while others seem likely but have yet to be proven beyond a shadow of a doubt. In particular, benefits such as lowered risk of irritable bowel syndromes and cancer-protective effects have been suggested by laboratory and clinical tests in Europe and Japan but have yet to be verified by thorough double-blind studies on both animals and humans. Some of the needed research is already under way, while some of it still waits to be done.

1. Boosting the Immune System

A number of studies show that two different types of organisms which commonly occur in yogurt, *Lactobacillus bulgaricus* and *Streptococcus thermophilus,* can bind to human T lymphocytes with high frequency and to B lymphocytes with low frequency (lymphocytes are cells that are involved in the production of antibodies needed to fight infectious diseases). This may provide one explanation of how yogurt and other probiotic foods can enhance immune function, helping the body to resist infections. These bacteria also adhere to the walls of the intestines, helping to maintain a healthy IM and to stimulate the activity of immune cells within the bowel environment. Animals that are fed *L. bulgaricus* and *S. thermophilus* show increased proliferation of lymphocytes, stimulation of B lymphocyte response, and activation of macrophages (cells that "eat up" and destroy invading organisms). In petri dishes, human peripheral blood lymphocytes were able to produce 3 to 4 times as much gamma interferon (a substance that inhibits viruses) than normal when a small amount of cultured yogurt was added. Finally, *L. bulgaricus, S. thermophilus,* and other lactic-acid producing bacteria have shown the ability to migrate to Peyer's patches (special intestinal immune tissue) and lymph nodes associated with the intestines, where they stimulate the body's immune responses (De Simone, et al., 1988).

2. Inhibiting the Growth of Pathogenic Organisms

Probiotic bacteria inhibit the growth of pathogenic organisms by successfully competing for available nutrients in the intestines.

They also inhibit pathogenic organisms by forming a sort of "living wallpaper" that covers the inner lining of the intestines. This effectively covers up the binding sites on the walls of the intestines that pathogenic organisms need in order to "get a hold" in the body and start growing. (When pathogenic organisms succeed in gaining access to these binding sites, they can multiply at an alarming rate, eventually outnumbering beneficial species. That is why infection by pathogenic organisms in the intestines—as with *Candida albicans*—is called *overgrowth* or *superinfection*.)

Also, probiotic bacteria have been shown to play a role in the production of antibiotic chemicals such as bacteriocins, which are deadly to other species of bacteria, and volatile fatty acids, which act as food for the intestinal mucosa (or lining). Thus, they increase the body's resistance to "colonization" by pathogenic organisms (Nord, 1984; Hentges, 1986).

3. Preventing Diarrhea from Various Causes

A number of studies have shown that adding *Lactobacillus acidophilus* to milk products can increase their digestibility and decrease diarrhea and other unpleasant digestive symptoms, such as gas and bloating, that often result from lactose intolerance (Hill, 1986). Also, one study found that administering a fermented milk product containing live *L. acidophilus* cultures helped reduce diarrhea in women who were receiving radiation treatment for gynecological cancer (Salminen, 1988).

4. Cancer Prevention

Some researchers have estimated that 80-90% of all cancers are the result of environmental factors and are thus preventable

(Drasar, 1974). Since the lining of the digestive tract has a huge surface area, it gets a great deal of exposure to potentially harmful external influences such as carcinogenic pesticides, synthetic chemicals, and even *naturally* occurring toxic compounds (such as those found in many foods). Thus it should be no great surprise that some studies indicate the IM may play a major role in preventing bowel cancer (Gorbach, 1990). Incidentally, according to a tremendous body of modern research, the best way to avoid bowel cancer (and probably other types of cancer as well) is to eat a whole-foods diet low in fat, meat, and sugar, and high in fiber (Wilkins and Tassell, 1983).

Interestingly, probiotic organisms may also help prevent breast cancer. A recent study showed that increased consumption of cheese and milk-fat was correlated with a higher incidence of breast cancer, while increased consumption of yogurt (which presumably contained lactobacilli or other probiotic organisms) was linked with decreased risk of breast cancer (Le, 1986).

"Interestingly, probiotic organisms may also help prevent breast cancer."

---

5. Reducing the Risk of Inflammatory Bowel Disease

Inflammatory bowel diseases, such as colitis, Chrohn's disease, and irritable bowel syndrome, may be linked with an unhealthy intestinal microflora. It has been suggested that acute inflammatory bowel disease transforms into chronic inflammatory bowel disease only when the IM is of a certain composition (Hill, 1986).

6. Improving Digestion of Proteins and Fats

By fermenting protein- and fat-containing foods, probiotic organisms increase the absorbability and thus the effective nutritional value of these foods. For instance, researchers have found that dried yogurt had a gross protein digestibility value of 94.5 compared to 85.0 for plain skimmed milk (Hasseltine & Wang, 1986; Reed, 1983).

7. Vitamin Synthesis

Many types of intestinal bacteria can synthesize some vitamins. However, we do not yet know for sure whether these vitamins are produced for the needs of the bacteria themselves or for the benefit of the host (i.e., us), or both. At any rate, it is known that intestinal bacteria can synthesize the vitamins B1, B2, B6, B12, folic acid, and biotin, among others (Drasar, 1974).

8. Detoxification and Protection from Toxins

Ammonia: During the digestive process, a number of toxic compounds are created in the body, one of the most harmful being ammonia. Ammonia is the form of nitrogen most toxic and readily absorbed by the body; it is produced in the intestines during the digestion of food (especially protein). People who eat red meat frequently are likely to have higher levels of ammonia in their blood than vegetarians, and they are more likely to suffer bowel cancer. However, fermentation caused by the IM decreases the duration and intensity of the intestinal mucous membranes' exposure to free ammonia by breaking it down with certain enzymes. Also, increased fiber consumption and supplementation with *L. acidophilus* or other probiotic microorganisms can help reduce the harmful effects of ammonia (Visek, 1978).

Cholesterol: The IM can break cholesterol down into a number of byproducts. It has been shown that a normal person can excrete up to 800 mg/day of cholesterol and cholesterol byproducts. In one test with human volunteers, a cholesterol-lowering effect was noted with a 1-week addition of cultured yogurt to the diet (Shahani, 1983). Because cholesterol has been linked with heart disease and colon cancer, the conversion of cholesterol to the nonabsorbable byproduct coprostanol may be a very significant factor in reducing overall body cholesterol levels (Hill, 1986).

Human Hormones: Hormones such as corticosteroids, progesterones, androstanes, and estrogens are all deconjugated, reduced, and dehydroxylated by cultures of normal human IM. Thus the IM may act as an important regulator of steroid hormones in the body. This has important health implications, since abnormally high levels of estrogens have been implicated in some types of cancer, as well as pre-menstrual syndrome (PMS).

9. Potentiation and Deactivation of Medicinal Substances

A number of glycosides from common medicinal plants, such as the active anthraquinone glycosides in senna and amygdalin in wild cherry bark, are activated or inactivated by the enzymes beta-glucosidase and other glycosidases produced by the IM. Thus the IM helps mediate the medicinal effects of certain naturally occurring substances. (Since it is beyond the scope of this book to review all the studies that have been done on the

IM's effect on glycosides from foods and herbs, interested readers are referred to Drasar, 1974 and Goldman, 1983).

10. Providing Energy for the Intestinal Mucosa (Lining)

The intestinal mucosa, or inner lining of cells, derives about 70% of the energy it needs from the short-chain fatty acids produced as a byproduct of bacterial fermentation in the IM. Thus the IM is indispensable for maintaining the health and reproductive vigor of the cells that compose the intestinal lining (Hill, 1986).

11. Maintaining Proper Mucus Levels in the Intestines

In some experiments, animals with very low IM bacterial counts showed five times greater mucus concentrations in parts of their digestive tracts than animals with flourishing IM systems. Since it is known that the IM breaks down mucus to get energy, it thus seems likely that the IM has an important regulating effect on the thickness and composition of the intestinal mucous barrier (Heneghan, 1973). This is significant because many health specialists have expounded a "mucus-free diet" over the years. The theory behind this recommendation is that a thicker mucus layer will inhibit the exchange of nutrients and the elimination of wastes through the colon wall. Milk, refined sugar products, and other "junk foods" are often said to be mucus-forming, and therefore they are to be avoided. Hopefully future studies will determine how much mucus should be present in the intestinal tract and will clarify the role the IM plays in maintaining these levels.

Microflora Formation in Infants

The formation of the IM begins at birth. As the infant passes through the birth canal, she or he is "inoculated" with microflora from the mother's vagina (Midtvedt, et al., 1988). Later, breast-feeding provides bacterial and immunogenic substances that create a simple flora of bifidobacteria, a genus of beneficial lactic-acid producing bacteria especially common in babies. Significantly, studies show that a formula diet can allow potentially pathogenic bacteria, such as clostridia and anaerobic streptococci, to proliferate in an infant's digestive tract. It has also been found that the addition of cow's milk to a baby's diet can decrease the numbers of bifidobacteria in the intestines and increase the pH and numbers of bacteroides present—neither of which are desirable (Drasar, et al., 1986). Thus, once again, so-called "improvements" over breast-feeding may not be improvements at all!

Recent research suggests that the composition of the IM established by the end of infancy greatly affects the composition of the IM later in life (Alm, et al., 1983). Drasar (1974) has drawn the conclusion, based on his research and that of others, that the composition of the IM is extremely flexible up to the age of weaning on to solid food, but that thereafter it becomes less adaptable. The delicate process of the creation of a probiotic microflora within the infant's intestinal tract, as well as the IM's full impact on health, may become better understood in the future.

Negative Side Effects of Antibiotics

There is no question that antibiotics are invaluable medicines. In emergency situations—such as in the case of a child on the verge of death from meningitis—antibiotics are literally lifesavers. Even in many less extreme situations, they may help keep people with serious or chronic infections alive. Nonetheless, antibiotics are too often overused in current medical practice, causing marked negative side effects, one of the greatest being damage to the intestinal microflora.

The negative effects of antibiotics on the IM have been extremely well researched. Freter, Bohnhoff, and others conducted pioneering research on this subject in the early 1950s. This early work has since been confirmed and augmented by many others during three decades of research. For a good review of the scientific literature published on this topic to date, interested readers are referred to Hentges (1986).

> *"The main problem with antibiotics is that they kill bacteria indiscriminately—the bad as well as the good."*

The main problem with antibiotics is that they kill bacteria indiscriminately—the bad as well as the good. This is, of course, not much of an issue with small applications of topical antibiotics. But with extended treatments of oral antibiotics, it can be a real problem. For instance, it is well known that broad-spectrum antibiotic treatment quickly reduces the numbers of beneficial organisms in the intestines, mouth, and vagina. The effect on the IM is of special interest here. As antibiotics that are incompletely absorbed or broken down in the small intestine reach the large intestine, they destroy many kinds of probiotic organisms there. Even relatively small doses (1/100 of the therapeutic dose) have been shown to severely disorder the function of the IM (Gustafsson, 1983).

The effects of a weakened IM, for reasons explained previously, can be quite detrimental. Once probiotic organisms have been destabilized and stripped off the walls of the intestines, potentially pathogenic organisms such as *Candida albicans*, staphylococci, and *Clostridium difficile* have much more opportunity to proliferate. This can lead to infection, sepsis, diarrhea, and colitis (Hill, 1986). Significantly, these conditions usually coincide with a reduction in the number of *L. acidophilus* in the intestines (Lidbeck, et al., 1988).

In the 1960s, there were a number of reports of people developing acute staphylococcal enterocolitis after treatment with broad-spectrum antibiotics, especially tetracycline (Drasar, 1974). Lack of similar reports today may reflect a change in the normal IM towards greater resistance. However, this does not mean that the normal IM today is invulnerable to the negative side effects of long-term antibiotic treatment!

A second major side effect of antibiotics is that they can lead to the emergence of antibiotic-resistant strains of bacteria. For instance, the important pathogenic bacteria *Shigella dysenteriae*, *Clostridium difficile*, and *Klebsiella* sp. have all been known to develop resistance to a number of antibiotics, which has made treatment increasingly difficult over the years. Up until 1954, *Shigella dysenteriae* could be treated easily with sulphonamides, streptomycin, chloramphenicol, or tetracycline. Now, however, strains that are resistant to all of these antibiotics, as well as to ampicillin, are common (Nordbring, 1983).

Fortunately, research on probiotic organisms is suggesting new ways to deal with the problem of antibiotic-resistant strains of bacteria. For example, in one study of infants who were being given ampicillin, supplementation with *L. acidophilus* organisms prevented superinfection by antibiotic-resistant strains of bacteria. In another study, concerning *Candida albicans* overgrowth in the intestines of four people taking the antibiotic clindamycin, it was found that *L. acidophilus* supplementation caused the *Candida* to disappear in three of the subjects. The researchers concluded that their findings "may indicate that the administration of *L. acidophilus* can reduce the risk of *Candida albicans* infections in compromised patients" (Lidbeck, A., et al., 1988).

The conclusion one should draw from the research cited is not that antibiotics should be discarded, but that their use should be minimized. Also, when their use is essential, it is best at least to combine them with probiotic supplements to maintain the IM. Below I explain five simple steps to take to reduce the risk of side effects from antibiotics. See page 72 for a discussion of the negative side effects of antibiotics.

As a final note, I should point out that other drugs besides antibiotics have been shown to alter the normal IM. These include anticancer drugs (chemotherapy), immunosuppressive agents (for preventing rejection of foreign tissue in organ transplants), and histamine H2 antagonists. If you are taking such medications, you might try a good probiotic supplement containing a variety of species (see the recommendations concerning using supplements at the end of this chapter).

Ways to Minimize the Side Effects of Antibiotics

1. **Avoid unnecessary use of any antibiotic.** Diet, herbal remedies, fasting, vitamin and mineral therapy, hydrotherapy, and rest are natural ways to eliminate infections without resorting to antibiotics. Antibiotic therapy should be the last resort. If you absolutely must take antibiotics, follow the other suggestions below.

2. **Use antibiotics for as short a period as possible.** After the acute phase of an infection has passed, discontinue the antibiotics, if possible, and use holistic treatment protocols instead. The damage to the IM will be minimized if the antibiotic treatment is limited to only a few days. It may be best to take a higher dose of antibiotics for a few days than a lesser amount for an extended period. Knock out the main infection quickly and then restore the IM with fermented foods and probiotic microflora supplements. In chronic infections, there are always underlying imbalances that must be addressed; antibiotics may be necessary for a short period (3 or 4 days), but the root cause must be identified and eliminated for lasting success.

3. **Use narrow-spectrum rather than broad-spectrum antibiotics.** In other words, use antibiotics that attack a specific or limited range of organisms rather than ones that kill any and all bacteria. This may reduce the negative impact on the body's microbial ecology.

4. **Always take probiotic microflora supplements.** Many of these, including ones containing *Lactobacillus* sp., have been

shown to minimize the unwanted side effects of antibiotic therapy (Hooker and DiPiro, 1988).

Finally, please note that certain antibiotics are more likely than others to induce the growth of resistant pathogenic strains of bacteria, destroy beneficial species, and stimulate pathogenic bacterial overgrowth or superinfection. Generally speaking, many of the "third generation" and newer antibiotic drugs, such as third generation cephalosporins, have a high potential for causing these side effects. Fortunately, penicillin is one of the least problematic antibiotics, and should be chosen first, if possible, where allergy is not a problem. Among well-known antibiotics, penicillin shows a low risk for inducing superinfection, ampicillin a moderate risk, and erythromycin a high risk. For more information on this topic, see Hooker and DiPiro (1988).

Traditional "Cultured" Foods

History

"Cultured" foods are fermented foods that have some kind of bacteria, fungus, or other organism growing on or in them which enhances the food's flavor, digestibility, or nutritional value, and which acts as a preservative. Examples of traditional cultured foods (and drinks) from the regions of Europe, the Mediterranean, and the Middle East include yogurt, sauerkraut, kefir, olives, pickles, beer, wine, vinegar, cheese, cottage cheese, and buttermilk. Cultured foods traditionally eaten in certain parts of Asia include various soy sauces, shoyu or tamari, tempeh, mochi, amasake, and kim-chi, as well as beers and wines.

It is difficult to say how far back in history people first made use of cultured foods. Soured milk is frequently mentioned in the Bible, and "soured milk of kine and goat's milk" mixed with fat were mentioned by Moses as one of the foods given to his people by Jehovah. Leben raib, made from fermented goat, cow, or buffalo milk, has been eaten in the Middle East since antiquuity. Of course these references are from Judeo-Christian history. Fermented foods were also important in many other ancient cultures as well.

Benefits of Eating Traditional Fermented Foods

Fermented foods were useful in ancient times because they are naturally resistant to putrefaction, or spoilage. Today artificial (and not especially healthful) preservatives and refrigeration have all but eliminated fermentation as a means for preserving foods. Nonetheless, there are still many good reasons to eat cultured foods:

- They increase the digestibility of protein and other nutrients;
- They reduce the risk of illness due to contamination by pathogenic organisms (studies have shown that aflatoxins, naturally occurring substances that may cause liver cancer in humans, are entirely absent in a number of traditional fermented foods);
- They enhance the odor and flavor characteristics of food;
- They may increase levels of some important nutrients in foods, such as vitamin B12.

Following is complete information on how to make two popular cultured foods, sauerkraut and yogurt. For information on how to make other types of fermented or cultured foods, see Hesseltine and Wang (1986) in the Resources list in the Appendix.

Sauerkraut

Sauerkraut has many medicinal properties. It acts as a laxative and antibacterial agent; protects against ulcers and bowel cancer; and promotes weight loss. Here's what you'll need to make this wonder food:

√ A large stone crock (1-5 gallon) that is glazed inside, with a tight-fitting lid
√ Organic cabbage
√ Flavoring herbs (juniper berries, rosemary, thyme, etc.)
√ Knife, shredder, or Cuisinart
√ A thermometer and pH strips

There are several ways to make sauerkraut, but the basic steps are always the same. First, finely shred organic green cabbage using a knife, shredder, or Cuisinart. Place the shredded cabbage into a large stone crock that has been sterilized with boiling water. This crock should be glazed inside. Crush the cabbage down to form a 1-2 inch-thick layer, and pour on a little cabbage juice prepared with the aid of a juicer. Sprinkle on any desired herbs or small amount of salt. This is now your first complete layer. Repeat this procedure to form subsequent layers until the crock is filled to within 2-3 inches of the top. Then cover the last layer with a few clean, washed cabbage leaves and place the cover on the crock. It is important to exclude air from the fermenting kraut, since undesirable organisms such as *Pseudomonas, Flavobacterium, Acinetobacter*, molds, and oxidative yeasts will readily grow in the presence of air and will spoil the batch or at least lead to an inferior product. Therefore, make sure to cover it with a tightly-fitting lid and weight the cover down with a couple of clean bricks or stones (about 6 pounds or so).

As the kraut starts to ferment, the pH should drop from 6.2 to 4.2 within the first 48 hours, indicating the formation of lactic acid. After two more days, the pH should drop to 3.7. Maintaining the correct pH level is critical. You can purchase pH strips to monitor the level of lactic acid being produced at most drug stores. When measuring the pH, draw off a small sample of the brine with a sterile utensil and quickly close the lid again so that airborne microbes will not get in. It is also helpful to monitor the temperature closely. Keep the temperature between 70 and 80 degrees F. (20-27 deg. C.).

Another thing you should do every few days is open the crock and carefully remove any scum that has formed on the top of the cabbage with a sterile utensil. Then wash the lid and weights (if they are wet) and quickly replace the cover. When the scum ceases to form, probably after 3-4 weeks, the fermentation process is finished, and the sauerkraut is ready to eat. Pack your finished kraut into sterile glass canning jars and store in the refrigerator. The kraut should last for several months.

Tips: To fine-tune the taste, texture, and bouquet of your sauerkraut, try adjusting the salt content to between 1 and 3%. A salt content of less than 1.8% leads to a softer product, while over 3.0% gives a fibrous, tough product. For instance, if the batch is started with 5 pounds of cabbage, add between 0.8-2.4 oz of salt total. Also, other vegetables can be added to the cabbage, such as shredded or thinly sliced carrots, beets, cucumbers, onions, and tomatoes. Sea vegetables such as wakame, nori, kelp, and sea palm also make an excellent addition and enhance the nutritional value of the kraut. Likewise you may add a variety of herbs to enhance the flavor and medicinal properties of your sauerkraut, among them juniper, rosemary, thyme, ginger, and lemongrass.

Yogurt

Like sauerkraut, yogurt has many medicinal properties. It improves digestion and the absorption of fat and proteins; provides high levels of essential amino acids; increases the production of B-vitamins; and it contains more assimilable forms of minerals, such as calcium.

"Yogurt has earned the right to its reputation as an outstanding medicinal food."

Pliny, a Roman historian writing in 76 B.C., recorded the use of fermented milk products for the treatment of a number of gastrointestinal infections (Reed, 1983). Today, after millennia of folk use and many modern scientific studies, yogurt has earned the right to its reputation as an outstanding medicinal food. Eating correctly made yogurt on a regular basis may help alleviate or even eliminate inflammatory bowel disease (colitis and irritable bowel syndrome), constipation, diarrhea, overgrowth of pathogenic organisms after antibiotic therapy, gum inflammation, elevated cholesterol levels, lactose intolerance and allergic reactions to dairy products, and liver disorders associated with increased levels of ammonia in the blood. Because lactose is consumed by the lactic-acid producing bacteria used to make yogurt, many lactose-intolerant individuals may eat yogurt (as wells as cultured milks) without suffering gastrointestinal upset. And finally, yogurt may also prevent and possibly aid in the treatment of bowel cancer (Reed, 1983).

Here are some guidelines and recommendations for making healthful yogurt.

Heating — Begin by placing goat, sheep, or cow's milk in a stainless steel or glass sauce pan. This milk should be of high quality, i.e., it should be fresh, pure, and free of antibiotic residues and all other unwanted substances. (Unpasteurized, unhomogenized goat or sheep's milk is the most healthful.) Then, at the lowest heat obtainable, let the milk evaporate until about 75-80% of its original volume remains. Ideally this should take an hour or two.

In making a commercial yogurt product, the milk is usually heated to about 80-90°C for about 20-30 minutes. The heating destroys undesirable microorganisms. It also changes the chemical makeup of the milk, which improves the coagulation and consistency of the finished product by enhancing the gel characteristics of the yogurt and reducing separation of the whey. For home preparations of yogurt and similar products like kefir, it may be best to heat the milk enough to reduce its original volume by 15-20%, without actually simmering or boiling the milk.

Starters — Let the milk cool, then add a suitable probiotic starter culture. Commercial preparations use *Streptococcus thermophilus* and *Lactobacillus bulgaricus*, which are both available in health foods stores. Yogurt starters containing a variety of other organisms may also be available. However, the best method is to inoculate each new batch of yogurt with a bit of the previous batch. After doing this for four or five generations of yogurt, a natural environmental inoculum of lactic-acid producing bacteria will result in the cultured product. If a batch ever develops a foul odor and fails to coagulate properly, throw it out,

Probiotic Organisms in Fermented Dairy Products

There are a number of lactic-acid producing microorganisms that thrive in milk and give it its sour flavor: *Lactobacillus helveticus, L. casei, L. plantarum, L. bulgaricus, L. lactis, L. fermentum, L. acidophilus, Streptococcus lactis, S. cremoris,* and *S. thermophilus,* among others. *Leuconostoc cremoris* also does well and produces lactic acid, acetic acid, and alcohol. Of these, the three most widely used in commercial preparations are *Lactobacillus bulgaricus, L. acidophilus,* and *Streptococcus thermophilus.* It is noteworthy that *L. bulgaricus* produces fermented milk products with the highest lactic-acid content: 1.7% for *L. bulgaricus,* as opposed to 0.9% for *L. acidophilus* and 0.8% for *S. thermophilus. L. bulgaricus* is also a major producer of acetaldehyde, especially when in the presence of *S. thermophilus,* which itself makes an important contribution to the flavor of a good yogurt.

In any given fermented product, the dominant organism depends upon the kind of milk, the duration of fermentation, and the environmental conditions. For instance, *Streptococcus thermophilus* is dominant at 37°C, while *L. bulgaricus* becomes dominant at 43-45°C, giving a more sour product.

sterilize any containers, and start over.

It is well known that different mixtures of probiotic bacteria produce varying amounts of polysaccharides, which greatly affect the texture and coagulating capacity of the final product. If you don't like the texture or gel of a particular type of homemade product, try other strains of bacteria.

Texture and Flavor Enhancement — In commercial preparations, texture and flavor are regulated by adjusting the total fat and non-fat solid content. A fat content of 4% gives a sweeter and creamier product. When the fat content is lower, the non-fat solid content can be increased by evaporation, making for a texture and flavor that most people will prefer. If the non-fat solid content is increased too much, however, the finished product may taste grainy. On average, milk from cows has 3.34% fat, human milk (4.38%), goat (4.14%), and sheep (7.00%) fat content (Ensminger, et al., 1983).

In many countries, yogurt manufacturers are allowed to add thickening agents like gelatin, pectin, starches, and alginates (from seaweed). When certain mineral ions (like calcium) are too low, the coagulation of the yogurt is affected, so 0.02-0.04% calcium chloride can be added. This is calculated by multiplying 0.0002 to 0.0004 times the weight of the milk (approximately 2 pounds or 908 gms/quart of milk). It is best to work in grams, because it is such a small amount. For instance, if one were making 1 quart of yogurt, which would weight 908 grams, multiply 0.0002 x 908 to get 0.18 gms, or 180 mg of calcium chloride.

Crushed or blended fruit, honey, and other sweeteners can be added to the final product as taste dictates. However, note that these may cause gas and bloating in some susceptible individuals.

Incubators — A variety of commercial yogurt incubators are available, including small cups that are placed on a warm plate or holder, a quart-sized warming electric "thermos," and others. One can make a suitable incubator from a small box and a light bulb. Some people make yogurt in their oven using the gas pilot to keep the temperature at about 38-45°C. I used to make yogurt and buttermilk on the top of a hot water heater enclosed in a small closet, because this environment happened to provide a perfect temperature for this purpose.

Cooling — Exactly when and how quickly an incubating yogurt is cooled controls the acidity and thus the sour flavor of the product. The fermentation process usually doesn't take more than 16-24 hours, and longer fermentation times will usually result in a product that is quite sour, which may be more therapeutic but is usually less palatable. The cooling process also initiates the "cold gelation" of the curd, determining the texture of the product. If the cooling is begun too soon, the flavor will be weak and the texture poor, possibly leading to separation of the whey. Commercial producers generally wait for the pH to reach 4.70-4.50, and then cool the yogurt to about 6-8° C., as quickly as possible, using refrigeration.

Storage — Note that all fermented milk products are sensitive to sunlight. Thus direct exposure to sunlight should be minimized during incubation and storage. Fermented dairy products should be refrigerated (in glass bottles or jars) to slow down bacteria growth and preserve nutrients.

Contaminants — Bacterial, yeast, or fungal contaminants are all possible in yogurt. None of these is known to be harmful, but they may lead to the presence of "off" flavors, odors, or an undesirable final texture in the finished product. Fortunately, many lactic-acid producing bacteria also produce substances (such as hydrogen peroxide) that inhibit the growth of contaminants. Thus, as long as you use fresh, high-quality raw milk and a healthy probiotic starter, there should be little problem with undesirable contaminants overgrowing in the final product.

Here is a list of some other substances (called bacteriocins) generated by probiotic organisms, other than hydrogen peroxide, that can inhibit undesirable contaminants:

Organism	Bacterial Product
Streptococcus lactis	nisin
Lactobacillus brevis	lactobrevin
Lactobacillus plantarum	lactolin
Lactobacillus bulgaricus	bulgarican
Lactobacillus acidophilus	acidophilin

Commercial Yogurt Products

A few words about commercial yogurts: Although supermarket shelves are lined with numerous brands of yogurt, it is doubtful that these products are especially healthful or that they really add any probiotic organisms to one's diet. Why? Well, first of all, most of the commercially available products contain refined white sugar, corn syrup, or some other concentrated sweetener. All of these are best avoided, given that for many people even moderate consumption of these sweeteners can lead to immune suppression and weaken the adrenal/pancreatic/thyroid axis (or cause kidney yin deficiency in TCM).

Secondly, commercial yogurt products often contain stabilizers such as gelatin, an animal product derived from mostly unhealthy cows. Also, the milk used in these products comes primarily from unhealthy cows that do not graze on open range, but rather are fed synthetic feeds fortified with chemical nutrients, antibiotics, and steroids to increase milk production and reduce sickness (which is often prevalent in the wretched environment these animals are forced to live in).

Finally, as a general rule, pasteurized cow's milk is for the most part unsuitable for human consumption—though fermentation probably improves its value by aiding assimilation of protein and other nutrients as well as reducing the possibility of allergies. The balance of calcium to other minerals in it is more suitable for a rapidly growing calf than for a human being. Also, after superheating and homogenization, the natural nutritional balance of the milk is irreversibly altered—many of

Fermented Alcoholic Drinks

Alcoholic beverages, when taken in moderate amounts—and preferably with a meal—may have beneficial properties such as increasing enjoyment of a meal, improving digestive function and assimilation of nutrients, improving blood circulation, and giving a sense of relaxation and well-being. (Alcohol abuse is, of course, not healthful.) Fermented alcoholic beverages may also be a source of beneficial microflora. However, to be so they must be processed very little after fermentation.

In this book no attempt will be made to review the procedures for making alcoholic beverages. For a good review of the history, uses, and preparation of traditional alcoholic drinks from a variety of cultures, see Gastineau, et al. (1979) and Darby (1979).

the protein chains are changed, making the milk potentially allergenic to some people. It is a fact that pasteurized cow's milk is one of the most common food allergens; it has been linked by many health writers to digestive problems (such as loose stools), chronic mucous-membrane infections, and inner ear infections, as well as to other health problems. Thus, healthy alternatives to supermarket yogurts are the brands of commercial yogurts found in natural food markets. Better still, make your own yogurt from certified raw cow, sheep, or goat's milk—as described above.

Using Probiotic Supplements

Now that you are more familiar with the benefits of probiotic microorganisms, you may be interested in trying commercial probiotic supplements, which are available in most natural food stores. Probiotic supplements are very popular in Europe and Japan, among other places in the world, and their use is growing in this country. Although you can get beneficial microorganisms by eating traditional foods such as sauerkraut, yogurt, rejuvelac, and others, in today's world there may be distinct advantages to adding a potent probiotic supplement to your diet. For instance, today we are commonly exposed to a number of pernicious environmental and dietary influences which may disrupt the normal balance of the IM, including:

- Chlorine and other bacteriocidal chemicals, which are often added to city drinking water;
- Chicken and other commercial meats that may contain residues of antibiotics given to animals to prevent infections;

- Pesticides and herbicides that may be present in various fruits and vegetables;
- Excessive sugar, fat, red meat, and refined foods, which may promote undesirable species of bacteria in the IM;
- Excessive raw vegetables, since these contain natural compounds which may inhibit the implantation of probiotics; and
- Alcoholic beverages, which also inhibit the implantation of probiotics.

Below, in question-and-answer format, I present the information that most people want to know when considering probiotic supplements. Be aware that since probiotic supplementation is still a young field of medicine, the experts do not always agree on what is best. However, there is already enough agreement to give some useful general guidelines. Part of this information is summarized from a symposium entitled "Probiotics: The Friendly Bacteria," which was held February 15, 1992 in Dallas, Texas. See the General Reference section for a list of presenters.

For what conditions should I take probiotics?

Following is a list of conditions and situations for which probiotic supplements may be useful. Note that you should ease into a probiotic program by taking 1/2 the recommended dose for a week or two. Also, when beginning a program of supplementation, you may have increased gas for a short while. This condition should disappear within a week.

1. **During antibiotic treatment:** As discussed previously in this chapter, antibiotics can disrupt and deplete the IM. Thus probiotic supplements are helpful. Begin by taking the recom-

mended dose of your probiotic product *before* you start the antibiotic therapy, if possible—otherwise start as soon as possible. Then take up to 2X the recommended dose during antibiotic therapy and return to the normal dose after the therapy is over.

2. **Constipation:** Long-term use of probiotics can help promote regularity.

3. **Diarrhea:** Short-term or long-term use can help prevent diarrhea.

4. **During pregnancy:** Probiotic supplementation during this important time can support your increased nutritional needs and promote bowel regularity. Supplementation during breast-feeding may also be helpful.

5. **Programs for infants and young children:** Supplementation with bifidobacteria is recommended, since these are the species of bacteria that infants and young children need most. These bacteria may help support the immune system, establish a strong IM, and protect against diarrhea and other bowel disorders.

6. **Counteracting infections:** Lactobacillus supplementation may help prevent recurrent urinary tract infections (such as cystitis). For gum and tooth infections, take your favorite probiotic supplement and rinse the mouth regularly with a solution made of 1 capsule of lactobacillus to 3 ounces of water. For vaginal infections (*Chlamydia, Trichomonas, Candida*) take a supplement containing lactobacilli and douche regularly with a solution of *L. acidophilus*, made in a 1:3 ratio as above. Finally, for chronic bowel infections any type of probiotic supplement may prove helpful.

7. **Irritable bowel syndrome:** Long-term use of lactobacillus or mixed-species supplements may help prevent irritation and

other symptoms of this syndrome.

8. **Chronic gas:** Gas is produced when bacteria in the large intestine work on starches, proteins, and other materials that are not broken down and absorbed in the small intestine. Bitter tonics and other digestive herbs are very beneficial for relieving this problem (see Chapter 5 for more details). A probiotic supplement may also be helpful to establish a healthier microbial balance.

What form of supplement is best?

Today probiotic supplements are available in several forms. The advantages and disadvantages of each are as follows:

Powder — Powder is convenient but is easily contaminated by measuring devices (spoons, etc.). It is also highly susceptible to the degrading effects of moisture and oxygen.

Capsules — This may be the best way to take probiotic supplements. Capsules are protected from contamination, oxygen, and moisture far better than powder.

Tablets — Tablets, like capsules, are also protected from contamination, moisture, and oxygen. However, the heat the microorganisms are exposed to during the tableting process may damage them.

Liquid — The problem with liquid supplements is that they are often weak and may contain few microorganisms. However, a fresh, high-quality liquid can be useful for douching and gargling. Some people find liquids more pleasant to take than capsules or tablets; if you are one, try opening a capsule or two and emptying the powder into a glass of distilled water. This will give you a more potent dose than a commercial liquid supplement.

Dairy — Today many dairy products are available that contain lactobacilli and other probiotic organisms. These products may be easier to digest for lactose-intolerant people, but they provide only a mild dose of probiotics.

When should I take the product?

The experts disagree—some say well before meals, some say after. In any case, what you *don't* want to do is take the supplement when your stomach is highly acidic, since strong acid kills probiotic organisms. Some experts feel that the food of a meal buffers stomach acid enough to make an environment acceptable to probiotic organisms. Others recommend taking probiotics between meals, when there is little acid in the stomach (Davenport, 1982). If this argument is true, then the *best* time to take probiotics would be in the morning, when stomach acid is at its lowest. In any case, it may be advisable to take a probiotic supplement with a little certified raw milk or some other dairy product (like your own homemade yogurt), since this provides food for the bacteria. Also, it is less effective to take probiotics after eating a lot of raw vegetables, because they contain substances that inhibit the bacteria.

How much should I take and for how long?

Take enough organisms to get the effect you want. Studies show that 6-10 billion organisms per day is generally appropriate for therapeutic use. This is usually equivalent to 2 or 3 capsules of the product per day. Probiotic supplements can be taken for several months, or even for years, if you feel they are of benefit.

What species are best? Is a mixed-species product better than a single species one?

The main species used are *Lactobacillus acidophilus, L. bifidus, L. casei, L. plantarum, Bifidobacterium bifidum, Streptococcus faecium,* and *L. rhamnosus,* among others (Sandine, et al., 1972; Speck 1976). Of these, *Lactobacillus acidophilus, L. bifidus, Streptococcus faecium,* and *Bifidobacterium bifidum* have been most studied in the laboratory. This is one reason why these latter species appear in products more than other species; another reason is because they commonly occur in some traditional fermented foods. In any case, every species of microorganism has different characteristics and effects; information on some of the most common species is presented at the end of this chapter. However, just because some species haven't been studied extensively doesn't mean they may not be valuable. In Table 10 I list a number of potentially healthful probiotic organisms that are common in traditional fermented foods. This information is summarized from the existing scientific literature on the subject.

Now regarding the question of whether single- or mixed-species products are better, the answer is up in the air. The issue is quite controversial. But since the experts disagree so much on this point, I think it is wisest to look to nature and the long history of traditional cultured foods until further scientific research is conducted. That is why, again, I think the species listed in Table 10 seem promising for supplementation. I would also point out that most cultured foods contain not a single species but rather a variety of microorganisms. For example, more than 100

Table 10
Most Common Probiotic Species
in Traditional Fermented Foods

Lactobacillus casei	(kishk, sour milks)
L. plantarum	(pulque, sour milks, sauerkraut)
L. pastorianus	(poi)
L. casei ssp. *rhamnosus*	(cheese, dairy products)
L. delbrueckii	(poi, koji)
L. leichmanii	(sorghum beer)
L. brevis	(sour milks)
L. bulgaricus	(jalebies, an Indian fermented bread)
Streptococcus lactis	(poi, sour milks, dahi)
Streptococcus kefir	(poi)
S. faecalis	(dahi)
Lueconostoc mesenteroides	(ambali and kimchi, Jalebies)
Rhizopus sp.	(tempeh, bakhar, chiu-chu, ragi, and many other foods, especially traditional Chinese fermented foods)
Aspergillus oryzae	(chu, soy sauce)
Pediococcus cerevisiae	(koji)
Pediococcus halophilus	(soy sauce)
Saccharomyces cerevisiae	(pulque)
Bacillus subtilis	(kishk)
B. megaterium	(kishk)
Agrobacterium azotophilum	(pozol)

species of microorganisms have been isolated from German rye sourdough bread. This emphasizes that our knowledge is limited--we have just begun to explore the rich microflora that lives in the fermented foods millions of people commonly eat every day. Also, it is known that the predominant species in a given cultured food will vary greatly depending on the starting materials used, the climate (especially temperature), and the specific conditions in which it is produced.

Can I trust the product to deliver what it says on the label?

No, not necessarily. Commercial preparations of *L. acidophilus* have long been thought to be of uneven quality (Probiotics Conference). A recent survey of 159 products of various types found that 70-90% of them contained fewer microorganisms than claimed; that liquid acidophilus products had almost no acidophilus in them; and that 1-2% of encapsulated/powdered products had no acidophilus in them (Shahani, Probiotics Conference). In short, when commercial products are tested, many fail to deliver the numbers and strain(s) of microorganisms, as well as the potency, promised on the label.

The moral of the story is: *always ask a probiotic company for full documentation on its product!* Don't feel hesitant to do this. Tests by independent labs should be available from the manufacturer proving that its product has the organism(s) stated on the label; that the organism(s) can implant in the human colon; and that the organism(s) produce the enzymes, lactins, lactic acid, and other substances advertised. If you need help contacting a manufacturer, ask the owner of the store where the product is sold; it is his or her responsibility to help you get the information you are requesting. Also, as a general policy, you shouldn't even consider a product that doesn't clearly state the date of manufacture, the base used (whether lactose or non-dairy), the species present, and the potency.

Finally, as long as you're asking questions, find out whether the product you are considering contains strains of microorganisms that resist the strong acids in bile. Some strains of bifidobacteria and lactobacillus do, and again, you should be able to obtain documentation to that effect.

Should the product be refrigerated?

All products should be refrigerated (or frozen) after opening, regardless of what they say on the label. The only exception is products that contain mostly *Streptococcus faecium*, which is stable at room temperatures.

How long will the product retain its potency?

This depends on the species involved. Again, *Streptococcus faecium* is very stable and needs little refrigeration if it is manufactured properly. If a product contains lactobacilli or bifidobacteria, however, it should be refrigerated or even frozen. Refrigerated lactobacilli will usually show a loss of about 3% per month, and frozen lactobacilli will die at the rate of only 1-2% per month. In contrast, at room temperature they will lose 5% per month, which adds up to about a 30% total loss in 6 months. In fact, tests have shown that mixed-species products containing *S. faecium, L. rhamnosus, L. acidophilus, L. bifidum,* and *Bifidobacterium* sp. may contain nothing but *S. faecium* after several months (Bailey, 1992) For this reason *S. faecium* is the best when traveling and when refrigeration is not available.

Note that freeze-dried products last the longest of all. They can last for several months without refrigeration; for up to a year with refrigeration; and for 1-2 years in the freezer. Also note that products in nitrogen-flushed glass bottles will retain their potency on the shelf longer than products in plastic bottles, since the latter breathe and the former do not.

Characteristics of Common Probiotic Organisms

Different types of probiotic bacteria have widely different

properties. Some produce high levels of enzymes that can help break down proteins; others produce enzymes that break down fats; and yet others produce chemical substances that help inhibit the overgrowth of pathogenic organisms in the digestive tract. *Lactobacillus bulgaricus* and *Streptococcus faecium*, for instance, both produce chemicals that neutralize the action of intestinal toxins produced by pathogenic strains of *E. coli*. Certain lactic-acid producing bacteria, on the other hand, provide their beneficial effect by adhering to the walls of the intestinal tract and preventing virulent pathogens (such as *Vibrio cholerae*) from taking hold there. Thus, even if these pathogens are present in the intestines in great quantities, they cannot become established and cause infection (Reed, 1983).

"Lactose absorption is up to four times better when acidophilus is added to low-fat milk."

Following is information about the characteristics and specific physiological effects of some of the most commonly available species of probiotic organisms.

Lactobacillus acidophilus

This is a common anaerobic bacteria (i.e., it grows only in an oxygen-free environment) that inhabits the digestive tract, mouth, and vagina. Although *L. acidophilus* produces less lactic acid than most other probiotic organisms, it still produces enough to have a noticeable beneficial effect.

Acidophilus is now commonly added to commercial brands of milk available in supermarkets. This is because acidophilus has been shown to improve lactose absorption and reduce the negative effects of drinking milk for people with lactose intolerance. Several studies have shown that lactose absorption is up to four times better in lactose-intolerant people when acidophilus is added to low-fat milk. The beneficial effects take about a week to develop to their fullest extent, and they last for about a week after the acidophilus supplements in the milk are discontinued (Speck, 1983).

Another significant positive effect of adding *L. acidophilus* supplements to the diet is that this probiotic organism may help bacterial populations that produce enzymes (beta-glucuronidase and nitroreductase, among others) that turn bile and other substances into carcinogens or mutagens (Speck, 1983). Interestingly, this effect is more pronounced in people who eat a lot of meat or fat than in people who eat a primarily vegetarian or high-grain diet. One study found only a small decrease in intestinal levels of these enzymes among subjects given *L. acidophilus* while on a vegetarian diet. But among subjects on a meat and fat-rich diet, a two- to fourfold decrease was found. This change developed over a period of one to two weeks and persisted as long as the *L. acidophilus* supplements were continued. After the supplements were stopped, it took about four weeks for the enzyme levels to return to normal. Only human strains of *L. acidophilus* adapted for implantation in the intestine showed these effects (Gorbach, 1986b).

Other important properties and effects of *L. acidophilus* include:

- Moderate generation time (about 64 minutes)
- Moderate acid resistance
- Can reduce coliform bacterial counts (this is important for reducing intestinal putrefaction)
- Antagonistic to a variety of intestinal pathogens, including salmonellae, staphylococci, and others (Speck, 1983)
- Reduces activity of the fecal enzymes ß-glucosidase and ß-glucuronidase, which may be involved in catalyzing the conversion of procarcinogens into carcinogens (Ayebo, et al., 1980)
- Helps degrade nitrates and nitrites, which are toxic and provoke genetic mutations (Speck, 1983)
- May help lower blood cholesterol (Speck, 1983)
- Protects against radiation

As a closing note, keep in mind that *L. acidophilus* cultures have a low survival rate when they pass through a highly acidic stomach milieu, that is, below pH 3 or 4. Their survival rate is better in a less acidic environment (pH 4 to 6), such as occurs in the stomach after meals. Thus, it may be best to take acidophilus cultures with a meal. Taking the cultures with a buffering agent may also increase their survival rate (Pettersson, 1983). Surprisingly, even under good conditions only a small percentage of acidophilus cultures (as little as 1-3%) will make it through the stomach and small intestine all the way to the large intestines. Nonetheless, this is enough to strongly influence the microbial composition of the colon. According to my own experience, as well as the experience of other researchers, therapeutic numbers of acidophilus can be maintained in the large intestine only when it is taken continually, with no more than an occasional break of a few days to a week. One study showed that bacterial composition in the large intestines returned to pre-supplement levels within nine days of discontinuing the cultures (Lidbeck, 1988).

Lactobacillus bulgaricus

This is a transient species in the IM, that is, it is not a permanent resident of the digestive tract. *L. bulgaricus* is the main microorganism in commercial yogurt. It produces good quantities of lactic acid and contains the proven antibiotic bulgarican (Reddy, et al., 1983)

Lactobacillus casei ssp. rhamnosus

This species of lactobacillus looks a lot like acidophilus—the two have been confused in the past. Modern taxonomists have determined that many of the early studies on acidophilus were actually performed with *L. rhamnosus*. Yet the health-promoting qualities of *L. rhamnosus* may be superior to those of *L. acidophilus*. *L. rhamnosus* ferments 24 carbohydrates vs. 11 for acidophilus; it has a superior survival rate against stomach and bile acids; and it has a rapid generation time. *L. rhamnosus* also boosts immune response (Rogovin, Probiotics Conference).

Bifidobacteria

These bacteria are a genus of anaerobic bacteria that commonly inhabit the large intestine and vagina. They appear bifurcated or split at one end, hence the name *bifid*, which means "two."

Bifidobacteria, especially *B. bifidum*, are a major component

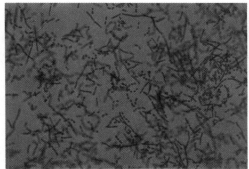

Lactobacillus bulgaricus and *Streptococcus thermophilus* are the most commonly used species of probiotic microorganisms used in commercial yogurt.

Lactobacillus casei ssp. rhamnosus looks a lot like *L. acidophilus*, but may become even more important commercially because of its rapid generation time and superior survival rate against stomach and bile acids.

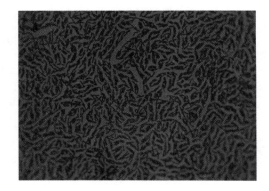

of the natural microflora of infants and children (up to 99% of a breast-fed infant's IM is made up of this single species), and breast milk contains high concentrations of bifidobacteria. It should be no great surprise, then, that several studies have shown that *B. bifidum* can protect infants against some intestinal infections. In one of these studies, it was found that a milk formula containing *B. bifidum* was helpful in preventing the overgrowth of *Candida albicans* following penicillin therapy (Rasic, 1983). Like other lactic-acid forming bacteria, *B. bifidum* also breaks down lactose, thus increasing lactose tolerance. It also improves the absorption of protein and minerals such as calcium. For these reasons, bifidobacteria are often added to cow's milk as a dietary supplement for infants and children.

"B. bifidum is probably most effective when combined with L. acidophilus."

Bifidobacteria are also important for the elderly, who are prone to developing bowel problems, such as diarrhea and painful digestion. These problems are often the result of a deficiency of lactic-acid producing bacteria in the intestines, whose job it is to protect against potentially harmful and putrefactive bacteria, such as enterobacteria, clostridia, and enterococci.

A further negative effect of the proliferation of putrefactive gut bacteria is that they can produce potentially toxic compounds (including ammonia). These toxins are normally detoxified in the liver before being excreted in the urine and feces. However, if the liver is congested or diseased and cannot detoxify these compounds properly, they can enter the bloodstream, eventually reaching toxic levels in the brain. To minimize the risk of such problems at any age, but especially among the elderly, who may be more sensitive, reduce the dietary intake of protein (particularly animal protein) to not more than 40-50 gm/day and add regular probiotic supplements to the diet. Note that for adults, *B. bifidum* is probably most effective when combined with *L. acidophilus,* since the adult small intestine has higher concentrations of lactobacilli than bifidobacteria. Thus fermented milks containing both acidophilus and bifidobacteria are recommended. However, the strongest therapeutic agent for the elderly, if tolerated, is pure cultures of these bacteria in lactose. Since these latter supplements are less effective when the diet is too rich in meat proteins, again it is recommended that elderly individuals reduce their intake of animal proteins.

Following are other key properties and effects of bifidobacteria:

- Produce acetic, lactic, and formic acids, which lower the pH in the large intestine and thus inhibit the growth of undesirable bacteria
- Can synthesize thiamine, riboflavin, vitamins B6 and K, and possibly other vitamins as well
- Help prevent and eliminate intestinal infection in adults as well as infants, especially when taken with lactulose
- Can lower blood levels of toxic compounds such as ammonia, free phenols, and indican
- May stimulate a positive immune response when taken

regularly

- May positively influence the metabolism of amino acids
- May assist protein metabolism in patients with liver cirrhosis (Rasic, 1983)

Streptococcus faecium

This beneficial organism is a normal component of the healthy colon. It is a type of enterococcus (group D streptococcus) that produces large amounts of lactic acid. Its characteristics and advantages are as follows:

- Reproduces rapidly (generation time is about 20 minutes)
- Exhibits good acid resistance
- Shows good resistance to many types of chemical antibiotics
- Is heat-resistant—it can survive for many months at 90° F.
- Produces bacteriocins, or antibiotic substances that are active against a variety of pathogenic organisms, including *E. coli*, *Salmonella*, and *Listeria*
- Reduces blood levels of ammonia in patients with severe liver diseases
- Can help prevent overgrowth of bacteria after antibiotics
- Persists up to a week after supplementation is discontinued
- Found naturally in cottage cheese and other dairy products
- Several commercial products have been available in Denmark (Paragurt®), Italy, and Japan for over 70 years.

One of the key uses of *S. faecium*, supported by many studies, is in the treatment of diarrhea, especially when it is a side effect of antibiotic therapy (Lewenstein, 1979). In one study, 104 patients between 1 month and 9 years of age were treated for diarrhea caused by enteritis (inflammation of the intestines) or antibiotic therapy with a special strain of freeze-dried *S. faecium*, SF68. For comparison, the subjects were split into two groups, one of which was given *S. faecium*, while the other was given a preparation of freeze-dried *L. acidophilus*, *L. bulgaricus*, and *Streptococcus lactis*. The subjects given *S. faecium* showed a much faster recovery from diarrhea—62% after two days as compared to only 35% for the control group. The researchers concluded that *S. faecium* shows greater natural antibiotic properties and growth rate than *L. acidophilus* (Bellomo, et al., 1980).

These findings were confirmed and amplified a year later by a controlled double-blind study conducted in Italy. In this study 29 patients with acute enteritis were given either an antibiotic consisting of bacitracin and neomycin, or a preparation of a particular strain of SF68. At the end of the treatment period, only 69% of the antibiotic group were "cured" as compared to an impressive 93% of the probiotic group. Remarkably, even after only 48 hours, the group given *S. faecium* cultures showed a 56% cure rate, while only 31% of the antibiotic group were cured by that point (Camarri, et al., 1981). As a result of these studies, in Denmark preparations containing freeze-dried cultures of *S. faecium* mixed with small amounts of other streptococci and lactobacilli are now recommended by health practitioners as protection against diarrhea during treatment with tetracycline (Friis-Møller, 1983).

Other studies have shown that *S. faecium* also provides protection against vitamin deficiency, which often occurs as a result of long-term antibiotic treatment. Furthermore, one study found that *S. faecium* protects against liver stress due to the consumption of antibiotics or alcohol, and it also reported that blood levels of ammonia—another cause of liver toxicity—were reduced with the use of *S. faecium* (Borgia, et al., 1982).

Chapter 5

Herbal Therapy

Medicinal herbs traditionally have been and still are used by the majority of people in the world for prevention of disease and restoration of health. Nine hundred million Chinese people rely on herbs for a major part of their health care. In the United States, herbs have been largely supplanted by chemical drugs, but their use is becoming increasingly widespread due in part to the new awareness of personal health.

Medicinal herbs generally work in two major ways. First, they provide nutrients and elements that the body requires to carry out its basic processes. Secondly, they add agents which would not otherwise be found in the body, but which stimulate, relax, strengthen, or "fine-tune" the body's processes and abilities.

Herbal Energetics—An Overview

There are four major classes of medicinal herbs which are described below. A knowledge of these classes is important in understanding how to use a particular herb or herb formula—for what type of individual, under what circumstances, how much, and for how long.

1. Tonics

Tonics help maintain tone throughout the body—on the

106

cellular level, and ultimately the tissue and organ level. "Tone" is a state of dynamic equilibrium, or balance, in the body or a part of it. Many substances and experiences can act as tonics, like a brief cold shower, but here we will focus on herbal tonics. Herbal tonics are very gentle and slow stimulants, and they provide nutrients that the body can use, such as vitamins, minerals, and perhaps many other types of essential compounds. These include plant pigments like anthocyanins or flavonoids or plant sterols. Large quantities of tonics can be given without risk of overstressing cells, tissues, or organs, because the therapeutic and toxic doses for tonics are very far apart. In other words, there is a large margin of safety.

I further divide tonics into two major subdivisions.

Stimulating tonics: These herbs and foods act to stimulate and invigorate bodily processes or parts. For instance, bitter herbs such as gentian or artichoke stimulate all the digestive processes, as long as they are not used excessively by the individual who is taking them. Stimulating tonics usually taste bitter, acrid, or spicy. Examples are gentian, golden seal, and other bitter herbs, as well as bitter greens (i.e., dandelion, kale, and endive), which are both nutritive and bitter.

Nourishing tonics: These herbs and foods supply important nutrients that cells, tissues, and organs need for proper functioning. They are usually sweet-tasting and considered foods. Examples are the herbs astragalus, codonopsis, jujube dates, lycii berries; and traditional foods such as yams, tapioca, poi, taro, gobo, aduki beans; and superfoods such as nettles, barley greens, spirulina, and chlorella.

Tonics are remedies that are well-tolerated, slow acting, do not force the body to change, and have a nourishing, strengthening, and normalizing effect on body systems. Tonics should be taken for at least 3 months, up to one year or more.

2. Specifics

These herbs are moderately active stimulants that must be given in lesser amounts and for shorter periods than tonics; otherwise over-stimulation and unwanted side effects may occur. Specifics are remedies that gently move or "adjust" a process in the body, whether it be hormonal, nervous, or related to immune function. Thus they are catalysts or assisting remedies. Specifics generally work by stimulating a process. One of the best examples here is echinacea, which stimulates macrophage function and thus confers heightened resistance to pathogenic influences (infections). Specifics are ideally used only as needed, usually for up to two or three weeks at most, though they can also be used in small amounts for longer periods, in which case they become more tonic-like. The therapeutic and toxic doses for specifics are closer than for tonics, but there is still a good margin of safety in most cases.

3. Heroics

These herbs are strong, irritating, and cause dramatic changes to occur. They must be used very carefully, because the toxic and therapeutic doses are very close. Certain heroic herbs are toxic, but when used properly for a very short time can "blast" through congestion or stagnation in the body. Examples of some heroic herbs are foxglove (digitalis), belladonna, and nux vomica (strychnine).

4. Protectors and cleansers

These herbs and substances remove wastes and pollutants from the body. Some do not materially affect the actual processes of the body, like bentonite clay taken in water solution, while others may interact with immune sensors or other body mechanisms. Examples of the latter type of protectors and cleansers are ionic substances such as pectin, as well as other soluble and insoluble fibers. Also, certain plant pigments, such as flavonoids, simply accumulate in the tissues near the skin and thus help protect against damage from ultra-violet light, but these have other pharmacological effects, too, such as protecting blood vessels.

Besides having the energetic qualities just described, medicinal plants also have an affinity for certain organs and organ systems (i.e., dandelion for the liver), and they have certain medical and traditional actions. The actions of herbs that especially affect the liver and digestive system are summarized in Table 11. Finally, in Traditional Chinese Medicine (TCM), the energetic qualities of herbs are said to derive from their tastes. Each flavor is said to have a particular effect on the body. These are summarized in Table 12.

Table 11
The Main Classes of Digestive and Liver Herbs

Class	Action	Herbs
Astringents	increase nerve and muscle tone; drying; remove moisture; can reduce bacteria, yeast, or viral overgrowth	oak bark, twigs, and galls (oak apples); blackberry root; black walnut
Bitters	stimulating; tonify nerve supply to digestive organs; increase flow of secretions and enzymes	dandelion, mugwort, wormwood, gentian, cascara sagrada, bitter orange peel, unripe apples, pears
Demulcents	cooling; soothing; relaxing	marshmallow root, slippery elm bark, flax seed, almond seed, barley
Anti-spasmodics	regulate chi; remove congestion	wild yam, chamomile, yarrow, passion flower, California poppy, fennel, peppermint
Anti-inflammatories	heat-clearing	chamomile, licorice, Oregon grape, golden seal, plantain, fenugreek, feverfew, meadowsweet, willow bark, poplar buds
Aromatics, carminatives	cool interior and warm surface, such as mucous membranes; smooth flow of chi; help release gas; relax sphincters; increase bowel peristalsis	peppermint, spearmint, fennel, caraway, dill, sage, lemon peel, orange peel, cardamon
Laxatives	stimulate and regulate the bowels, usually when there is lack of bowel tone, or constipation. Herbs with a very mild laxative effect are called *bowel tonics*, and very strong laxatives, *purgatives*	rhubarb, cascara sagrada, aloe, senna, buckthorn

Table 12
The Flavors in TCM

The Five Flavors

Sweet

Nourishes cells; supports wei chi (immune protective vitality); tonifies the digestive system and blood

Salty

Balances cellular function (especially movement of substances into and out of the cells); excess amounts increase moisture, while a deficiency of salt can dry, depending on the situation; mineral salts support nerve function

Sour

Removes and counteracts toxins; balances pH; affects nerve transmission; stimulates activity of digestive enzymes and liver; astringent

Acrid

Moves energy; supports assimilation; increases transformation of yin to yang; penetrates to interior of digestive, respiratory, and urinary tracts

Bitter

Small amounts stimulate and moisten yin, increase digestion (assimilation, elimination), enhance immune protective function; larger amounts are drying, contracting; stimulates liver function

The Three "Flavor Qualities"

Aromatic

Cools interior and warms surface (i.e., mucous membranes); smooths flow of chi (immune and vital energy)

Demulcent

Cools and soothes surface (mucous membranes); calms overactive immune force locally (useful for allergies); active in respiratory, urinary, and digestive tracts

Astringent

Contracts and dries, especially the mucous membrane system in the bowels, upper respiratory tract, and urinary tract

How to Make Herbal Teas

Home preparations of herbs are often made by simmering the fresh or dried herbs in water. For flowers, leaves, and other light herbal parts, make an infusion by bringing water to a boil, taking it off the heat, adding the herbs, and then covering and letting the mixture steep for 10 to 20 minutes. For heavier herb parts— such as roots (slices or cut and sifted pieces), bark, and seeds— make a decoction by actually simmering the herbs for 20 minutes to one hour.

To judge how much herb to add to a measured amount of water, use the general formula of 1:10 for decoctions and 1:20 for infusions, where the 1 is one part of the herb by weight (grams or ounces), and the 10 or 20 is the water by volume (milliliters or ounces). The ratio of herbs to water, as well as the length of time for cooking or infusing, can be varied according to need and taste. The longer an herb steeps, the stronger the tea. However, sometimes the nature of the preparation will change if more of the less-soluble components (such as tannins) go into solution. Thus, if a peppermint tea infusion is left in the pan to infuse overnight, the astringent taste becomes increasingly pronounced.

Finally, it is best to prepare herbs in a stainless steel pot, glass coffee pot, or traditional ceramic or clay pot. Strictly avoid teflon-coated pans or aluminum. Herbalists agree that these may act as a source of potentially toxic substances or affect the energetic properties of the tea.

Dosages: How much of an herb or herb formula is given is almost as important as its intrinsic nature. In practice, one will often find that a small amount of a specific herb or herb combination is tonic, more of it will be specific, and even more can be toxic. Even though large amounts of a tonic herb or herb formula in theory should not become specific, in practice they may become so after protracted use.

The average maintenance dose for an infusion or decoction is 1/2 to 1 cup morning and evening. The average therapeutic dose is 3 cups per day. Specific herbs are best taken in a cycle of 10 days on, 3 days off, 10 days on. Repeat this cycle 3 times total. Tonic herbs can be taken in the same cycle but for much longer periods of time (up to several years if profound weakness exists, as with AIDS).

To check for individual sensitivity and response when taking an herb or combination for the first time, start with a mild tonic dose for a few days, then gradually work up to a full therapeutic dose. When discontinuing a remedy, taper off over a few days, rather than cutting it off abruptly. This way the body is not shocked.

Evaluating Commercial Preparations

A wide variety of ready-made preparations are available in natural food stores, herb shops, and even supermarkets. Whenever possible, support your local natural food store. Often the supplement department has well-trained people to answer questions. At any rate, the service and support in holistic and herbal information will be much more reliable in a natural food store or herb store.

The main preparations to be found as finished products are the following:

1. *Powdered herbs in capsules.* These are fine for mild

complaints and may be taken up to 2 to 4 capsules 2-4 times daily.

2. *Liquid extracts (tinctures)*: These are fine for mild to moderately severe complaints. They are concentrated and hold their potency for up to 3 years; are easy and convenient to use; and are fast-acting. A normal dose is 3 dropperfuls per day, taken either in the morning, afternoon, and evening each, or 2 in the morning and 1 in the evening.

3. *Powdered extracts*: These are fine for mild to moderately severe complaints. They are much more concentrated than simple powdered herb products and have a 3-year shelf-life under optimum conditions. They are also potent and moderately fast-acting and are good for people who want an alcohol-free preparation. An average dose is 3 tablets or capsules per day.

When selecting a product, make sure to choose a company that uses organically-grown herbs in their products, where available. If a company has many organic herbs in their line, it is more likely that the overall freshness, identity, purity, and quality will be superior as well. The quality of the herbal product is probably the single most important factor determining its effectiveness. Ask the store supplement consultants, if in doubt. Always read the label to find out whether the company uses high-quality herbs (the label should read *certified organically-grown*), whether the herbs are in powdered form or in extract form, and the amounts of each herb present. Also, compare with other brands to check for value. For example, if a bottle of echinacea has 90 capsules of simple herb powder at a size of 400 mg per capsule, this would be the same as 90 capsules of herb concentrate (1:4) at 100 mg.

Judging a tincture is not so easy, but generally a 1 ounce bottle of liquid extract may equal a 90-count bottle of herb capsules of 400 mg each. However, because liquid extracts are easier for the body to absorb, it is likely that the immediate effect one will experience with the liquid will be greater.

While the form of the herb can be significant in determining dosages, it is the quality (freshness, identity, purity, and potency) of the original herb that went into the product, one's consistency in taking the product, and one's receptivity to the remedy that determine the ultimate outcome. This is, of course, assuming that a correct evaluation or diagnosis of one's constitution and condition has been made in the first place and that the prescribed herbs are the right ones for the conditions.

Bitter Tonics or "Bitters"

In the traditional medicine of both Europe and China, bitter herbs are thought to tonify and strengthen not only the digestion, but the whole nervous system and vital energy of the body as well. Bitter tonic formulas, often called "bitters" in Traditional European Medicine (TEM), usually contain bitter herbs like gentian, golden seal, artichoke, angelica, or blessed thistle, plus some aromatic or spicy herbs, such as ginger, fennel, or cardamon, to help counteract the tendency of the formula to cool and contract the digestive tract in some people. Many ready-made bitter formulas are available in natural food stores and even in grocery stores and liquor stores (angostura bitters), though when they come from the latter two sources, they must be checked for sugar and other undesirable additives.

Bitters are still used extensively in many cultures to strengthen

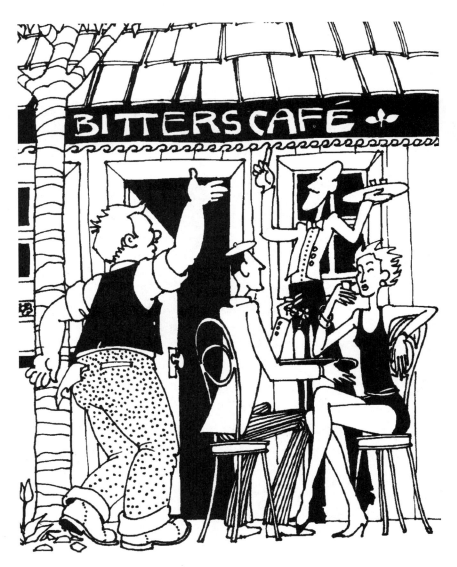

digestion. For example, in Europe, "bitters cafes" are a popular
social stop on the way home from work, because they are
thought to prime the digestive tract for the evening meal.

European naturopaths regularly recommend bitter wild greens or small doses of unripe fruit (such as green apples) to increase the digestive powers. When I traveled in Greece, I was delighted to discover that small, unripe, sour and bitter plums are eaten before meals. One sees vendors with pushcarts selling them in many places throughout the country.

In some cultures, wild greens, or salads, are eaten before the main meal. For instance, in Greece I also witnessed people collecting and consuming wild chicory greens in large quantities. Like many of the wild greens I discussed in the chapter on Diet Therapy, wild chicory greens have mild bitter principles that activate the digestive juices and thus prepare the body to digest the proteins, fats, and carbohydrates that follow. A little lemon juice or vinegar on the greens adds a sour taste that has been shown to improve assimilation of iron, zinc, and other elements and to activate the liver. All of the traditional practices described above make good sense, since by reflexive nerve action the bitter flavor immediately activates the secretion of juices and tonifies the digestive muscles. Research shows that the bitter constituents of some herbs powerfully activate and strengthen various aspects of digestion as well as of other body processes, including nerve function. Some of these bitter compounds, such as amarogentin in the herb gentian, are so powerfully bitter that they can be detected in a dilution of 1:50,000.

To summarize the research to date, bitters work in three major ways:

1. They **activate the gastric secretion of hydrochloric acid** and of other digestive enzymes, such as bile. This increases the nerve tone of the muscles in the entire digestive tract and improves blood circulation, thus enabling the body to utilize

foods, absorb nutrients, and eliminate wastes more effectively.

Interestingly, in one study it was discovered that bitters can activate gastric secretions by directly stimulating sensors in the stomach, not just through taste receptors and nerves in the mouth. This is significant because, although bitters may work best by using a liquid preparation where one can actually taste them and thus have saliva production increased, they will also have an effect when swallowed in capsule or tablet form.

2. They **increase the strength and tone of the autonomic nervous system**, which supplies nerve force to (or energizes) all the digestive organs without our thinking about it consciously.

Bitters may also be helpful in lowering anxiety and counteracting stress. Our autonomic nervous system is made up of two opposite branches—the sympathetic (flight or fight) branch and the parasympathetic branch. One can relate the sympathetic with the yang, outgoing, functional side of our being, and the parasympathetic with the yin, nutritive aspects. While strengthening digestion, bitters activate the parasympathetic branch of our autonomic nervous system, or the metabolism of nutrient substances, which is called in TCM, "gaining yin and consuming yang" (Yanchi, 1988). Most people living in industrialized countries are usually in a constant state of "gaining yang and consuming yin," which is a poetic way of saying that we are over-extending ourselves and are stressed out. Bitter tonics, then, may be a great way to help restore yin-yang balance.

3. They **activate the immune system**. Recent studies show that some bitter herbs, such as gentian, can modulate the gut-associated immune system. This is extremely interesting, given that one of the main indications for bitter formulas in Europe is for people recovering from infectious diseases, including viral-

based disorders such as chronic fatigue syndrome. Also, when the intestine is affected by a chronic inflammatory ailment, such as irritable bowel syndrome or candidiasis, it is likely that an "auto-immune" inflammatory response is occurring, causing cramping, pain, scarring, and reduction of bowel function. If this overreaction can be lessened and balanced, then the problem can be resolved. For instance, clinical tests in Europe (Maiwald, 1987) have shown that bitters can decrease levels of sIgA antibodies and reduce or eliminate symptoms in people with inflammatory bowel disease.

When to Use Bitters

Bitter formulas are especially indicated for digestive weakness and pain that comes during or after infectious disease, which can deplete the vital energy of the body. Decreased vitality is insidious because if the absorption of nutrients and elimination of wastes is reduced, then the immune system and other systems of the body will suffer further. Indeed, many cases of indigestion—whether attended by pain, gas, or constipation or not—are directly or indirectly attributable to reduced vital energy. In today's world, increased population density and the competition that has arisen from it have helped create a situation where one must overwork to make ends meet. This stress can lead to depleted vital energy, which impairs digestion, which in turn further decreases the body's vital energy. Prolonged and intense mental work, especially, is depleting. People who use their mental faculties constantly and then have trouble "shutting it off" after work, run the risk of eventual mental and physical exhaustion, resulting in symptoms such as chronic fatigue, loss of appetite, loss of interest in life, and various aches and pains.

The following list summarizes the conditions for which bitters are used. For a list of important bitter herbs, see Table 13.

- Poor fat digestion
- Poor protein digestion
- Weakness due to chronic illness, especially when accompanied by viral or bacterial infections
- Loss of zest for life, lowered vital energy
- Painful digestion, intestinal cramps, excessive gas
- Irritable bowel syndrome
- Poor appetite
- Anemia, low hematocrit
- Excessive craving for sweets (my own observation)
- Immune-based disorders where nutritional deficiency is present
- Especially effective for digestive weakness due to mental overwork and lack of exercise

How to Take Bitters

It is important to recognize that bitters must be taken over a period of weeks or months before their full effect is achieved. Taking them for a day or two might bestow some benefits, but 90 percent of the effect builds up slowly. Bitter formulas are taken one half hour to 15 minutes before mealtimes or just after eating. Usually 1/2 to 1 teaspoon of the liquid extract preparation, 1 or 2 teaspoons of a bitters tea (drink it at room temperature, not hot), or 1 dropperful of a more concentrated bitter formula is sufficient. If worsening of symptoms occurs, reduce the dose by one half for a week. Some commercial bitters also have a mild laxative component, achieved by adding such herbs as aloe and senna. These should be avoided by people who have diarrhea or loose bowels. I have found that these kinds of formulas sometimes do not agree with people who are deficient or lacking vital energy.

For people who are recovering from illness and have painful and weak digestion, it is best to take the bitters and emphasize small meals of whole grain porridges (corn, oats, rice, and barley), which are easy to digest. Even children do well on this regime.

Here is a recipe for "classic" homemade bitters.

"Classic Bitters"

Powder the following dried herbs in a blender and add to either vodka, brandy, or wine:

artichoke (1 part)

gentian (1/4 part)

orange or *tangerine peel* (1 part)

cardamon (1/4 part)

ginger rhizome (1/4 part)

Macerate (let soak) for 2 weeks, shaking the jar every day. Press or squeeze the liquid out and filter (optional). Store in suitable glass containers or amber dropper bottles (available in drug stores).

To make a bitters tea, simmer the herbs for 30 minutes at 1 part of the herb mixture to 20 parts of water. Remember that this tea cannot be kept outside the refrigerator without fermentation occurring, and even in the refrigerator, it should not be kept for more than 3 days.

Table 13
The Most Important Bitter Herbs

Angelica root	Warming, slightly bitter; a member of the parsley family often used in bitter formulations
Artichoke leaf	The leaf of the familiar artichoke; tastes bitter and salty; is slightly cooling; activates the bile
Bitter orange peel	Commonly mixed with gentian to moderate its bitterness
Blessed thistle	Native to southern Europe; ancient liver and gallbladder herb
Cascara sagrada	Famous Native American bowel tonic
Centaury herb	Close relative of gentian; not a bitter itself, but commonly used in bitters
Gentian root	The most bitter herb of all; small amounts are used in many preparations
Goldenseal rhizome	A favorite native American bitter tonic; use moderately
Lemon peel	Aromatic, protective, and slightly bitter
Mugwort herb	A common wild plant in many parts of the world; a relative of wormwood
Wormwood herb	One of the most popular digestive herbs in Europe
Devil's Claw	Reported to be useful as an anti-inflammatory herb for arthritis, but studies are inconclusive; activates gallbladder; strengthening and steadying effect on the heart

Herbs that Benefit the Liver and Gallbladder

Herbs especially are recommended for their liver-protecting qualities, because they contain large quantities of vitamins, minerals, and other active compounds in easily assimilable forms.

Herbs (in combination with a whole-foods diet) are often considered by herbalists and other natural health practitioners to be superior to synthetic vitamin, mineral, and amino acid supplements, which the body cannot absorb so readily and which may interfere with the uptake and utilization of other vital elements.

Also, since certain herbs have antioxidant properties, they can protect against excess free radicals. Herbs are also an excellent source for flavonoids, which are coloring pigments in plants that can strengthen blood-vessels, act as antioxidants, and have many other beneficial effects. And last, but not least, recent studies show that herbs contain compounds that have enzyme-modifying effects, providing structural elements to some enzymes (Chang, et al., 1985). See Tables 14 and 15 for a summary.

Table 14
Natural Liver Therapy with Herbs

Cleansers:	**Protectors:**
burdock	milk thistle
dandelion root	garlic
yellow dock	schisandra
blue flag	bupleurum
Oregon grape root	**Antioxidants:**
Builders:	rosemary
artichoke	lemon balm
milk thistle	saffron
butternut	turmeric
oat	**Warm Stagnant Liver:**
Cool Liver Fire:	prickly ash
gentian	ginger
dandelion	

Table 15
Sources of Liver-Protecting Substances

Antioxidants	Stabilizing	Choleretics	Sulfur Sources	Enzymes
Herbs & Foods				
milk thistle	milk thistle		milk thistle	
licorice				
artichoke		artichoke		
ginkgo				
capillaris		capillaris		
skullcap				
			dandelion	
cabbage	cabbage		cabbage	cabbage
rosemary				
bilberry				
eleuthero				
schisandra				schisandra
chaparral				
garlic	garlic	garlic		

The next two charts present herbs for the liver and gallbladder and give their actions in both traditional Chinese and modern Western terms. Note that there are no herbs specifically for the gallbladder, while there are herbs just for the liver. However, the double-action herbs for liver and gallbladder together are especially stimulating to the bile and the health of the gallbladder.

Table 16
Herbs for the Liver and Gallbladder

Genus	Common Name	Energy	Chinese Action	Western Action
Achillea	yarrow	neutral	purges fire	anti-inflammatory, decongesting
Allium	garlic	warm	dredges liver	warms, opens liver, stimulates bile
Anemone	hepatica	cold	pacifies liver	soothes liver, tonic
Antennaria	pussy paws	warm	-	deobstruent
Arctium	burdock	cold	purges fire	liver imbalances, stimulates bile
Artemesia	mugwort	warm	dispels wind	jaundice, opens liver
Artemesia	capillaris	cool	cools fire	liver imbalances, stimulates bile
Avena	wild oat	neutral	-	stimulates nerve tone, nutritive
Berberis	barberry	cold	purges fire	anti-inflammatory, opens liver, bile stimulant
Centaurium	centaury	cold	clr damp heat	stimulates, cleansing, tonic
Chelidonium	celandine	cool	dredge liver	removes bile stones, increases phagocytosis
Cichorium	chicory	cool	dredges, cools	deobstruent, opens, tonifies
Cnicus	blessed thistle	cool	dredges, cools	stimulates bile, opens, cools
Cynara	artichoke	cool	dredges, cools	stimulates bile, opens, regenerates
Gentiana	gentian	cool	clr damp heat	opens, cools, stimulates bile
Inula	elecampane	warm	subdues yang	slows, eliminates fluid
Lavandula	lavender	cool	-	calms emotions, antioxidant
Raphanus	wild radish	neutral	-	digestive tonic
Rosmarinus	rosemary	cool	-	warms surface, dispels wind, antioxidant
Silybum	milk thistle	neutral	yin tonic	regenerates, protects, stimulates bile flow
Taraxacum	dandelion	cool	dredges, cools	deobstruent, opens, tonifies

Table 17
Herbs for the Liver

Genus	Common Name	Energy	Chinese Action	Western Action
Angelica	angelica	warm	moistens yin	dries, dispels gas, builds blood
Berberis	Oregon grape	cold	purges fire	anti-inflammatory, opens liver
Bryonia	bryony	warm	-	acrid irritant, stimulates
Ceanothus	red root	cool	clears damp heat	anti-inflammatory, cleanses lymph
Chionanthus	fringe tree	cool	subdues yang	jaundice; bile obstructions
Coptis	gold thread	cold	purges fire	anti-inflammatory, detoxifies, dries
Coriolus	polypore	neutral	moisten yin	dries, increases phagocytosis, immune strengthener
Dioscorea	wild yam	neutral	supports stomach/spleen	balances hormones, nourishes
Galium	cleavers	cool	clrs damp heat	diuretic, removes wastes
Hydrastis	golden seal	cold	purges fire	anti-inflammatory, opens, stimulates bile
Iris	blue flag	cool	-	warms surface, removes congestion
Larrea	chaparral	cool	-	warms surface, detox., deobstruent, antioxidant
Leptandra	black root	warm	dredges liver	stimulates liver, bile, glands
Linaria	toad flax	warm	dredges liver	jaundice, liver, skin diseases
Picraena	quassia	warm	-	small dose regenerates, tones
Rhamnus	cascara	cool	dispels heat	bowel stimulant, clears liver congestion
Sanguinaria	bloodroot	cool	-	warms surface, mucosa, stimulates bile
Schisandra	5 flavors berry	warm	supports yin	protects liver, adaptogenic
Scutelaria	skullcap	cold	removes heat	subdues liver yang
Xanthoxylum	prickly ash	warm	-	warming, deobstruent, regenerates

Herbs That Benefit the Stomach/Spleen System (TCM)

As explained in Chapter 1, the TCM stomach/spleen system plays a central role in the processes of assimilation (conversion of food to energy and body substance) and elimination. When this vital system is not working properly, symptoms of immune dysfunction, chronic fatigue, painful digestion, weight loss, gas and bloating, and diarrhea can result. In TCM, herbal remedies play a central role in restoring health and balance to the stomach/spleen system. The herbs in Table 18 are ones that have been used since antiquity, as well as carefully researched in the laboratory and clinic. See the reference list for books that explore their activity and uses in more depth.

Table 18
Important Stomach/Spleen Herbs in TCM

Chinese	Latin	Function
Fu Ling	*Poria cocos*	removes dampness, strengthens the spleen
Huang Qi	*Astragalus membranaceous*	tonifies spleen Qi
Bai Zhu	*Atractylodes ovata*	benefits Qi, strengthens spleen
Yi Yi Ren	*Coix lachryma-jobi*	removes dampness, strengthens spleen, stops diarrhea
Ginseng	*Panax ginseng*	strengthens the spleen and stomach
Dang Shen	*Codonopsis pilosula*	strengthens spleen Qi, nourishes fluids
Shan Yao	*Dioscorea opposita*	strengthens spleen and stomach
Da Zao	*Ziziphus jujuba*	strengthens stomach and spleen
Gan Cao	*Glycyrrhiza uralensis*	tonifies spleen Qi
Huang Jing	*Polygonatum sibiricum*	strengthens stomach/spleen

In TCM, formulas are often preferred over single herbs. The following three traditional formulas are sold in small amber glass bottles. They are arguably the most popular of the stomach/spleen tonics available from stores that sell Chinese herbs, as well as acupuncturists. The formulas can also be ordered by mail (check Resource section on page 290.)

Hsiao Yao Wan (*Bupleurum Sedative Pills*)

This formula is one of the most popular of Chinese patents because it helps to harmonize the liver and spleen, generally improving digestion and relieving symptoms of PMS, when they are due to stagnant liver Qi. The formula strengthens the spleen and nourishes the liver.

Dose: take 8-12 small pills 3 x daily before meals.

Curing Pills (*Kang Ning Wan*)

A most popular formula for nausea and digestive upset. The formula contains 15 or more herbs, including coix, magnolia bark, atractylodes, angelica, rice sprouts, hoelen, and mint. It is useful to help regulate the stomach, remove excess mucus, and for resolving invasion of wind in the stomach meridian, with flu-like symptoms. It helps remove symptoms such as nausea, intestinal cramps, headache, and diarrhea. Curing pills are also used to counteract morning sickness or motion-sickness.

Dose: take 1-2 small bottles as needed.

Ginseng Stomachic Pills (*Ren Shen Jian Pi Wan*)

Especially good for chronic spleen Qi (digestive vitality) weakness with symptoms of bloating, gas, pain, and irregular bowel movements. Useful for people who cannot gain weight.

Contains unripe citrus peel, orange peel, ginseng, atractylodes, barley sprouts, and hawthorn fruit.

Dose: take 6-10 small pills 3x daily before meals. Should be taken for several weeks—up to 5 or 6 months for best results.

Laxatives and Bowel Tonics

An area of healing where herbs really excel is in strengthening and cleansing the bowels. It has been known from antiquity that certain herbs can help the bowels move, even removing old, encrusted matter. If the bowels lose tone from too many refined foods, herbs can help exercise and strengthen them. Modern research shows that most bowel tonic and laxative herbs work by stimulating the bowel wall, increasing peristalsis, as well as decreasing the uptake of water from the fecal mass as it passes through the colon, leading to looser stools.

Laxative and bowel-tonic herbs fall into three main categories depending on their strength and scope of activity.

1. **Bowel tonics** have a very mild laxative activity. These herbs (such as cascara sagrada and yellow dock) are used for exercising and strengthening the bowel muscles. They are *tonic* herbs.

2. **Laxatives** increase the regularity of bowel movements. These herbs (such as aloe, senna, buckthorn bark, and butternut bark) can help stimulate a bowel movement during times of constipation. They are *specific* herbs.

3. **Cathartic herbs** strongly clean out the bowels, removing worms, some encrusted fecal matter, and anything that might be "hanging around." Many native peoples used cathartics as part of a spring cleansing program or to rid the body of pernicious

or toxic influences. Note that cathartic herbs (such as jalap and mandrake) are a bit too strong and unpleasant for most people and are contraindicated for those with weak constitutions or who are recovering from chronic illnesses. These fall into the category of *heroic* herbs.

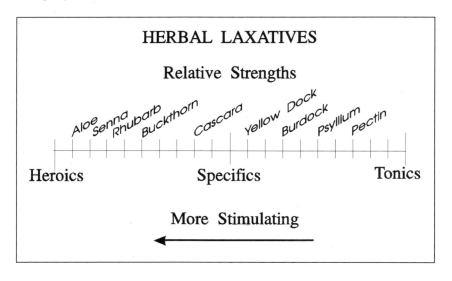

A large variety of bowel tonics and laxatives can be found in natural food stores, drug stores, and markets. Commercial laxatives should be avoided if they contain coloring, preservatives, or other chemical additives. If the bowels are very stuck and a strong laxative is desired, several herbs are available that will move the bowels, including senna, aloe, and rhubarb.

The bowel-tonic herbs can be used from several weeks to several months as part of a program to strengthen and regulate bowel function. Dr. Christopher's famous "Naturalax #2" is a good example. This formula contains cascara sagrada bark, barberry root bark, fennel seed, ginger root, golden seal, lobelia herb, red raspberry leaves, Turkey rhubarb root, and cayenne.

It is best to take laxative herbs for short periods only—i.e., for several days or up to 10 days at the very most. These are specific herbs that are used for the particular purpose of moving the bowels when they are stuck. Any other constipation or bowel irregularity should be dealt with by using bowel tonics and/or other natural methods over a long period of time. Here are a few natural methods that will help the bowels regulate themselves. These methods are time-proven and should give excellent results after a week or ten days. They should be practiced as regular living habits.

• **Never eat too late at night or too early in the morning**. The bowels should have a complete rest during the night. In the morning, make sure to have a period of activity of at least half an hour to an hour before eating breakfast. This gives the body a chance to "wake up." At night, stop eating at 6 or 7 pm, depending on your work schedule. Try not to eat anything but fruit or other light, natural snacks after dinner. If you crave food before bed, try drinking a cup of herbal tea with licorice.

• **Massage the lower abdomen** in a clockwise direction every day, working out any sore spots with your fingers.

• **Stop eating when full** or better, a little before.

• **Avoid eating** a big meal **when tired or upset**.

• A moderate **walk after big meals** will improve digestion and promote regular bowel movements.

• **Strenuous exercise** at least once a day **is excellent for the bowels**.

• **Eat plenty of high-fiber foods** at every meal.

• **Chew food well**.

For further information about intestinal and bowel cleansing programs see Chapter 6, pages 152-161.

Triphala

Triphala is an ancient Ayurvedic herbal formula consisting of three fruits, Amla or Emblic Myrobalan (*Emblica officinalis*), Bahera or Belliric Myrobalan (*Terminalia bellirica*), and Harra or Chebulic Myrobalan (*Terminalia chebula*). In India, it is used as a powder, as a jam, and as teas or other drinks (Dash & Junius, 1988), and commercial products are available in tablet form. Triphala is useful as a mild laxative and bowel tonic, promoting regularity and helping ease symptoms of gas and bloating after meals (Tierra, 1988), but it is considered a general strengthening and rejuvenating tonic in India, where it is also recommended for relieving asthma, bronchitis, diabetes, and obstinate urinary disorders (Dash & Junius, 1988). The dose is 2 tablets or 1/2 teaspoon of the powder 2 or 3 times daily.

Table 19
MAJOR LAXATIVE HERBS AND THEIR USES

Name	Constituents	Properties/Uses	Doses/Duration	Contraindications
Aloe *Aloe barbadensis* or *A. ferox*	anthraquinone glycosides: aloin (4.5-25%); free anthra-quinones: aloe-emodin; resins, gums, polysaccharides, steroids, saponins, etc.	one of the strongest bowel purgatives, used in stronger commerical laxatives; has also been recommended for hemorrhoids, jaundice, cirrhosis	for tonic effects, 30-120 mg; laxative effect, 120-600 mg of aloe resin	one of the most cramping of the laxatives; very bitter taste; best to take with ginger, cardamon, and other aromatics; habituating
Buckthorn *Rhamnus frangula* [aged at least 1 year]	3-7% anthraquinone glycosides, including glucofrangulin A & B, frangulin A & B, and various isomers of emodin; tannins, flavonoids, anthrones, and anthone glycosides	colon stimulant; very commonly used in Europe in commercial laxative products; a mild to moderate laxative—only mildly irritating, and though often added to bitter tonics, is less bitter than aloe or cascara; often used for chronic constipation	aqueous extract, 200-600 mg once a day; fluid extract (1:1), 1-4 dropperfuls; for chronic constipation, 1-5 grams in powder (3-10 "00" caps)	if used often, can sometimes cause mild cramping; if so, add aromatics like ginger or cardamon
Butternut bark	juglone, juglandin, juglandic acid and other naphtha-quinones; essential oil, tannin	for chronic constipation, poor bowel tone, and candidiasis, provided there is no diarrhea and only mild bowel irritation; stimulates bile, helps remove worms (use with garlic and black walnut); may aid hemmorhoids	tincture, 2-3 dropperfuls up to 2-3 x daily; 300-500 mg of the powdered extract; can be taken up to several months with care	like all laxatives, it can weaken bowel tone when used excessively, and cause mild griping unless used with aromatics

Cascara sagrada *Rhamnus purshiana*	maximum of 10% anthraquinone glycosides, consisting of nearly 70% cascarosides A,B,C, and D; resins, tannins	cascara bark must be aged at least one year, at which time it becomes an excellent mild laxative and bowel tonic for long-term use (up to several weeks or a month); specific for bowel peristalsis and chronic constipation; one of the most widely used bowel tonics—should be used with aromatics to counteract its cold and bitter nature	powdered bark, 1-2.5 g; 2-5 dropperfuls of tincture, or 100-300 mg of the powdered extract	because of its cold, bitter, potentially irritating properties, it should not be used by people who have cold or deficient spleen/stomach Qi
Castor oil *Ricins communis*	a number of fatty acids, especially triglycerides of ricinoleic acid (90%), as well as linoleic and oleic acids, and others	widely used throughout the world as a strong laxative and purgative; ricinoleic acid stimulates increased motor activity with little griping; copious liquid stools are produced about 6 hours after ingestion; is often used for removing intestinal contents in food poisoning	preferred dose is 4-16 ml—60 ml maximum in 24 hours	not recommended for use by people with deficiency states, especially spleen deficiencies; can cause intestinal irritation with large or frequent doses; can increase toxicity of some fat-soluble worm medicines
Psyllium *Plantago psyllium, P. indica, P. ovata*	both the husk and the whole seed are used; contains up to 30% mucilage-like polysaccharides, mainly in the husk; alkaloids, sterols, various fatty acids, tannins	one of the most popular bulk laxatives in world trade; many types of commercial preparations contain it; swells in the bowel when taken with sufficient liquid, expanding and stimulating the bowel wall as well as moistening and softening the feces; (cont.)	mix one teaspoon of the husk or seed powder into water and drink—always follow any mucilage-containing bulk laxative with ample liquid—preferably at least 1-2 glasses of water; psyllium can be used as needed for years, but should not replace proper (cont.)	though rare, the mucilage has the potential to stop up the digestive tract if not taken with ample liquid

Name	Constituents	Properties/Uses	Doses/Duration	Contraindications
		possibly beneficial in spastic, irritated colon, and constipation; may help remove toxins from the bowel; may have a cholesterol-lowering tendency; helpful for diarrhea	eating and bowel habits, such as eating a good variety of fresh fruits, vegetables, grains and legumes	
Rhubarb, Chinese *Rheum officinale, R. palmatum* Rhubarb, English *Rheum rhaponticum*	Chinese, English as well as Indian and Japanese rhubarb all contain various mixtures of anthraquinone glycosides such as emodin, rhein, chrysophanic acid, etc.; tannins are also important in rhubarb; calcium oxalate	English rhubarb is milder than Chinese; generally stimulates digestion, and is considered tonic, astringent, and mildly laxative; an important remedy in Chinese medicine; considered bitter and cold, it removes heat from the blood and bowels, detoxifies, relieves jaundice; indicated for "intestinal excess heat"; laxative effect is produced in 6-8 hours	3-6 grams in tea—do not boil for more than 10 minutes to avoid extracting too many tannins which increase its tendency to constipate in small doses	avoid during colds, flu, and other exterior conditions; avoid where there is deficient blood or Qi; best to avoid during pregancy and nursing; because of its cold nature, it is best to avoid in cold deficient spleen and stomach
Senna *Cassia senna, C. angustifolia*	the fruits and leaves are used; anthraquinone glycosides, mostly sennosides A, B, C, and D, and a number of others; mucilage, flavonoids, volatile oil, resins, etc.	one of the safest, and therefore one of the most widely used and predictable stimulant laxatives; used the world over for relieving constipation; taken by itself or with other laxative or aromatic herbs; often used in herbal weight-loss products	of the powdered leaves, 0.5-2 g; of the tincture, 2-4 ml (1-3 dropperfuls)	more than occasional use or excessively large doses can promote bowel weakness, laxative habituation, and eventually damage the bowel

Useful Digestive Herbs and Foods From the Kitchen

Cabbage
Cabbage juice is often recommended for ulcers of the stomach, esophagus, and duodenum. For this purpose, juice fresh green organic cabbage and drink about 6 ounces of the juice twice daily for 10 days on and 2 days off. It may take about 4 to 6 weeks before you notice improvement. It is important to be consistent and to reduce causative factors such as emotional and environmental stress, and stimulants such as coffee, tea, or chocolate, and especially soft drinks. Energetically, cabbage is sweet and demulcent and clears heat.

Chamomile
This is one of the most widely used digestive herbs in the world. Its use spread from Spain and Europe to the new world, and it can now be found in most outdoor markets throughout Mexico and Central and South America. Although many people consider chamomile a weak herb, it has powerful anti-inflammatory and antispasmodic properties when used in the proper amounts. Two primary indications are for nervous or irritable bowels, and colic in babies, children, and adults.
When taking chamomile, be consistent and drink substantial amounts of the tea. Try to find freshly-dried flowers that still have a nice golden color and are highly fragrant, rather than brown, old, scentless commerical herb. Make a tea by gently simmering 1 ounce of the flowers in 16 ounces of water for about 10 minutes. Let the decoction stand for about 20 minutes, then strain and store it in quart jars in the refrigerator. Drink a cup of the warm tea (with the addition of honey and a little fennel, licorice, or ginger) at least 3 times daily. In extreme conditions, you can drink up to 5 or 6 cups per day.
Since the most active compounds in chamomile are alcohol-soluble, a tincture, liquid, or powdered extract is stronger than a

tea. The therapeutic dose of these extracts is 120 to 500 mg of the powdered extract, or 2 to 3 dropperfuls of the tincture, taken 2-3 times daily. For maintenance after the symptoms disappear, take 1/2 of the above amount for an additional 7 to 10 days. Energetically, chamomile is aromatic, slightly bitter, and warming to the surface.

Caraway

Caraway is an excellent remedy to know about, because it is nearly always available during an emergency. It is a common kitchen spice, as are ginger and turmeric. Rudolph Weiss, a respected German herbalist and doctor, calls caraway "one of our most reliable and powerful carminatives". He also recommends it highly when combined with chamomile as a tea to help ease irritable colon. For this purpose, take 1 cup of the tea immediately after breakfast and lunch each and 1 an hour or two after dinner. The herb is often used to aid the digestion of fatty foods. Caraway is warming and enters the stomach and intestinal meridians.

Fennel

Like caraway, fennel is a seed from the parsley family. It is excellent for helping to remove gas and promoting good digestion. In Indian restaurants, one often finds a small bowl of fennel seeds at the cash register. Diners are supposed to chew a few of these seeds to remove the effects of dietary sins, such as overeating, wrong food combining, and eating excessive amounts of rich, spicy foods (like curries). Fennel is excellent for children, because it has a mild, licorice-like flavor. Mix a little licorice with fennel (1/4 part licorice to 1 part fennel), simmer for 20 minutes, let cool, and strain. Then give this tea to the child *ad lib* while fasting for painful digestion, colic, or diarrhea. According to Weiss, this will relieve intestinal spasms of painful bloating due to gas.

Flaxseed

Flax is the source of linseed or flaxseed oil, which is now being touted as an excellent source of essential fatty acids (linoleic and linolenic acids) that help relieve conditions such as arthritis, PMS, chronic inflammation in the colon, and auto-immune ailments. Because flaxseed is a food, it has a more tonic, normalizing effect in these cases than a specific would. Flaxseed and fennel are parts of the "Polari-Tea" that I often recommend as a cleansing tea (see recipe on page 145.) Flaxseed is demulcent and soothing, reducing irritation and inflammation in the mucous membranes, especially those in the colon and urinary tract.

Licorice

Licorice is so useful and revered in TCM that it occurs in more formulas than any other single herb. Modern science has shown it to have significant anti-inflammatory properties, and because of its sweet taste, it is used in candy and many food products. For medicinal purposes, use about 1/4 part licorice to other herbs, such as fennel and flax. However, remember that when licorice is taken in large amounts over an extended period, as when using the herb to help heal ulcers, it can increase the body's excretion of potassium and decrease elimination of sodium. Because of this, when taking significant quantities of licorice (more than 4 grams daily for 10 days), increase potassium supplementation and reduce salt intake. Licorice therapy is contraindicated for people with high blood pressure or those who are prone to edema, except under the care of a natural health care practitioner.

Peppermint

What herb could be more popular than peppermint? Its essential oil is used in everything from candies and bodycare products to soaps and toothpaste, as well as the ubiquitous after-dinner mint. What many people don't realize, however, is that peppermint has medicinal qualities. Peppermint tea is a wonderful preparation for children and adults to relieve pain due to gas or indigestion—fast.

Peppermint tea is usually available, even in chain restaurants, ready to help one through trying gastrointestinal times. But, just to be safe, always carry a small vial of peppermint oil in your purse or pocket. That way, if no tea is available, you can put one or two drops of the oil in a cup of hot water, stir well, and sip this "tea" to quickly relieve cramping and gas pains. Peppermint herb can be added to other herbal formulas to impart a pleasant, refreshing taste to the mixture, thus increasing the body's receptivity to the other herbs. Energetically, peppermint is aromatic, slightly bitter, and astringent.

Yarrow

This ancient plant, also called *Achillea millefolium*, was the herb of Achilles. As legend has it, the herb helped the great hero heal the wounds of his comrades in the battle of Troy. Be that as it may, yarrow grows wild in many parts of the world and is readily available to harvest either from field and coastal strand, or you may buy it from a natural food store in the bulk herb section. Yarrow has some energetic similarities to chamomile, plus a number of shared constituents. In addition, it possesses a good tonic bitter quality. Because of this, yarrow tea or other commerical preparations of the herb are useful for mild gallbladder or bile weakness, as well as for increasing bile secretion for detoxification or improved fat digestion. I consider this one of the best teas to take during saunas or sweats, as it increases elimination of toxic wastes. (See page xx for information about sweating therapy.) The classic yarrow sweating and detoxification formula is as follows:

> *Yarrow flowering tops (1 part)*
> *Peppermint tops (1 part)*
> *Elder flowers (1 part)*

Infuse the herbs for 20 minutes in boiled water, strain, and drink 1 or 2 cups as needed for colds, flu, or cleansing programs. Energetically, yarrow is bitter, mildly astringent, and cooling.

Chapter 6

Cleansing Programs

Throughout the ages, from Hippocrates (455 B.C.) to Norman Walker and Paul Bragg, healers and educators of natural health have all strongly emphasized the need to maintain a clean and pure state in all the systems of the body and spirit. In scientific terms, both metabolic waste products (internal toxins) and external chemicals with a potential for toxicity, such as over-the-counter drugs like aspirin and acetaminophen, have the ability to disrupt delicate enzyme systems, irritate and damage cells and tissues, and speed up the aging process. Hence various types of cleansing and detoxification therapies are healthful.

In this chapter we will explore eight major types of cleansing:

- blood purification
- lymphatic cleansing
- sweating therapy and other ways to improve elimination through the skin
- urinary cleansing
- intestinal and bowel cleansing
- the liver flush
- the gallbladder flush
- fasting

Blood Purification

Herbalists of old used the term *blood purifier* to describe an herb or formula that removed any kind of undesirable elements from the blood. Although somewhat nebulous, the concept of "impure blood" is certainly defensible within the modern view of human physiology. As a carrier of many kinds of necessary chemical substances, including hormones, local mediators such as prostaglandins, sugars, vitamins, and minerals, the blood also has the potential to hold undesirable substances such as pesticides, herbicides, viral particles, yeast cells, and bacteria. Today, a blood purifier can be defined as a substance or method (as in sweating therapy) that facilitates the elimination of wastes and toxins through the skin, kidneys, breath, and bowels. Blood purifiers also increase the activity and efficiency of the phago-cytes, which are immune cells that engulf and remove wastes and organisms from the blood and mucus.

The best herbs for blood purification are echinacea, yerba mansa, chaparral, red clover, burdock, yellow dock, sarsaparilla, and yarrow. The best nature-cure methods include sweating therapy (use a tea of yarrow, elder flower, and peppermint before and during); aerobic exercise; dry-brush skin massage; cold water therapy; juice fasting; and enemas. These methods are discussed in the following sections.

Lymphatic Cleansing

Lymphatic cleansing is often recommended during or after a chronic infection, when swelling of the lymph nodes, tumors, or cysts occurs. The lymphatic system carries the *lymph*, a nearly clear fluid containing proteins, wastes, and other elements. Lymph comes from the interstitial fluid that surrounds the cells of the body, and brings them nourishment and removes wastes. The lymph travels in the lymphatic vessels, which lie right next to the

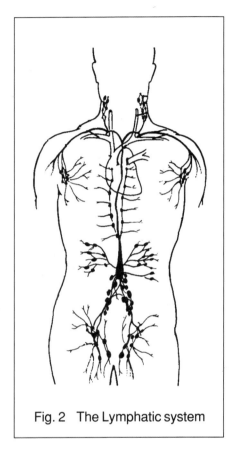

Fig. 2 The Lymphatic system

blood vessels and eventually connect back to major veins. Thus, in the end, the lymph flows into the blood system. Along the lymph vessels are located *lymph nodes*. These contain a high concentration of immune phagocytes that engulf and break down potentially toxic substances.

Unlike the blood system, the lymph does not have the luxury of a "heart" to pump it around. Instead, movement such as walking must "milk" lymph through the lymph vessels. Because of this, it is entirely possible to see a condition of stagnant lymph, especially when one has a sedentary life-style. After a winter of sitting inside and eating heartily to keep warm, the lymph can become very congested. For this reason, in the spring I often enjoy a lymphatic cleansing program consisting of a lymphatic massage and lymphatic cleansing teas.

For a lymphatic massage, oil your body well with a high-quality massage oil, and then "milk" or stroke the lymphatic channels, starting around your feet and ankles, then moving up to the calves, groin, and into the intestinal area. Then follow a similar procedure to move lymph down from the jaw, and through the neck, clavicle, breast area, and finally into the intes-tines. Of course it is not only more fun to receive a lymphatic massage from a friend or a professional therapist, it will probably be more thorough. There are lymph nodes in the body that are difficult to reach, even for the most flexible of people!

For maximum cleansing, fast for three days before the lym-phatic massage, or at least eat predominantly fruit. I also recommend the following herbal tea to be taken with or in place of the fast. Table 20 lists other good herbs for lymphatic cleansing.

Emphatically Lymphatic Tea

Red root (1/2 part)
Red clover tops (1 part)
Echinacea root (1/2 part)
Lemon peel (1 part)
Ginger (1/4 part)

Directions: Simmer 1 part of herb blend in 5 parts water for 20 minutes. Then strain and drink 1/2 cup of warm tea twice a day. A little honey can be added for flavor, if desired.

Table 20
Lymphatic Herbs

Common name	Scientific name	Comments
Red root (root bark)	*Ceanothus sp.*	one of the best-known and respected lymphatic herbs
Echinacea (root)	*E. purpurea* or *E. angustifolia*	activates phagocytes to help clean wastes from the lymph
Ocotillo (stem)	*Forquirea splendens*	a desert plant with a long history of folk use; an important lymphatic herb according to herbalist Michael Moore
Red clover (blossoms)	*Trifolium pratense*	contains saponins, coumarins, and flavonoids; a popular "alterative" for skin problems
Cleavers (herb)	*Galium aparine*	an excellent herb for reducing swelling of the lymph nodes; use internally, 40-60 drops of tincture 3x/day
Mullein (leaf)	*Verbascum thapsis*	contains saponins and mucilage; useful for activating the lymph circulation in the neck and chest
Figwort (leaf)	*Scrophularia nodosa*	traditionally used in both Europe and China to clear heat and reduce lymphatic swelling in the throat and neck
Prickly ash (bark)	*Xanthoxylum americana*	use with red root or other lymphatics to stimulate lymph activity, increase secretions, and help remove stagnation
Poke weed (root)	*Phytolacca decandra*	very strong lymphatic stimulant, especially in the breast and throat; use with caution externally and internally for lymph node swelling; works well in acute swelling or inflammation of the breast (acute mastitis) [Caution: this plant is toxic]

The Liver Flush

Liver flushes are used to stimulate elimination of wastes from the body, to open and cool the liver, to increase bile flow, and to improve overall liver functioning. They also help purify the blood and the lymph. I have taken liver flushes for many years now and can heartily recommend them. And if you make the herbal formula right, it can be quite tasty. Here are the instructions:

1. **Mix any fresh-squeezed citrus juices together** to make 1 cup of liquid. Orange and grapefruit juices are good, but always mix in some lemon or lime. The final mix should have a sour taste—the more sour, the more cleansing and activating. This mixture can be watered down to taste with spring or distilled water.

2. **Add 1-2 cloves of fresh-squeezed garlic, plus a small amount of fresh ginger juice**, which you can obtain by

Polari-Tea

Fennel (1 part)   Fenugreek (1 part)
Flax (1 part)   Licorice (1/4 part)
Burdock (1/4 part)   Peppermint (1 part)

Directions: Simmer the herbs for 20 minutes, then add 1 part peppermint and let the tea steep for an additional 10 minutes. For extra soothing properties, try adding 1/2 part marshmallow root (cut and sifted) to the initial tea blend.

grating ginger on a cheese or vegetable grater and then pressing the resulting fibers in a garlic press. (Note: Both garlic and ginger have shown amazing liver-protective qualities in recent studies (Hikino, 1986). Garlic contains strong antioxidant principles and also provides important sulfur compounds that the liver uses to build certain enzymes.)

3. **Mix in 1 tablespoon of high-quality olive oil**, blend (or shake well in a glass container), and drink.

4. **Follow the liver flush with two cups of cleansing herbal tea.** I like "Polari-Tea", which consists of the herbs listed on the preceding page. I make plenty of this tea and keep it in a quart canning jar, so it is always available.

Drink the liver flush in the morning (preferably after some stretching and breathing exercises), then do not eat any other food for one hour. This liver flush can be taken in cycles of 10 days on and 3 days off, as needed.

There are also several good commercial formulas for liver-cleansing available in natural food stores everywhere, both in bulk and in tea-bag form. One product I can recommend is a blend called "Puri-Tea" from herbalist Brigitte Mars. It contains peppermint, red clover, fennel, licorice, cleavers, dandelion, Oregon grape, burdock root, butternut bark, chickweed, parsley root, and nettles.

If you want more cleansing action than simple teas or formulas provide, try adding a fast with fresh fruit and vegetable juices. You can also take an enema each day. A good enema can be made by adding the juice of 1/2 of a lemon to 1 quart of tepid water (lemon-water in general is a good cleanser because citric and other plant acids in lemon juice can *chelate*, or bind with, and remove heavy metals and other toxic wastes accumulated in the body). Retain for 10 to 15 minutes (if possible), apply clockwise lower abdominal massage, then expel.

When and how often should one take liver flushes? I usually do two full cycles of 10 days on, 3 days off in the spring and again in the fall, with a 3-day rest between each cycle. However, I know many people who benefit from a single 10-day flush once at each equinox time. In any case, though, if one really feels a need for a liver flush, any time is the right time. I have never seen anyone experience negative side effects from this procedure.

The Gallbladder Flush

Please note: This technique is for people who have had previous experience with cleansing programs and have practiced a predominantly whole foods diet for some time.

The gallbladder flush is useful for people who are experienced with fasting and cleansing and who want to go a step further and remove even more old wastes stored in liver cells and other tissues. This flush should not be used more than once a year. I have seen some people become nauseated after drinking the flush, but nothing worse than that. Instructions follow.

1. About an hour before bedtime, drink 1/4 cup of extra virgin olive oil, followed by 1/4 cup of mixed, fresh-squeezed citrus juices (50% grapefruit juice, 25% lemon juice, and 25% orange juice). Repeat this process every 15 minutes for an hour, so that you drink a total of 1 cup of olive oil and 1 cup of citrus juice.

2. After the drinks, go to bed, making sure to lie on your *right* side. By tradition, this is thought to allow the oil to be discharged from the gallbladder more efficiently, but whether this is in fact true has not been proven as far as I know.

3. In the morning, take an enema consisting of 1 qt. of warm distilled water with the juice of 1/2 lemon.

Note: It is often good to combine the gallbladder flush with a 3- or 7-day juice fast. Toxic wastes released during fasting will be effectively eliminated during the strong bile flush and enema.

The purpose of this flush is to strongly activate the liver and gallbladder. When the liver encounters so much oil, it reacts by producing a large amount of bile, which the gallbladder then squirts into the intestines. It is thought that such a strong flow of bile will carry with it deeply stored toxins which are then flushed out of the body with the enema. Activating the liver and gallbladder so strongly may also run them through a thorough drill, thus strengthening them.

During the enema, watch for little green "stones" that may be eliminated. I have heard these called gallstones, but they are probably saponified oil. My own experience with the flush, plus my observation of others who have done it, has convinced me that old, negative emotions can be eliminated during the process. Anger and frustration, especially, are purged. It is possible that one may experience strange feelings during the process, as if some drug were in the blood stream. This may be due to old drug residues being re-experienced as they are eliminated from the body—or it may be due to a systemic hormonal reaction to all the oil. I tend to believe the former theory, but there are no definitive tests to prove which view is right.

Sweating Therapy

Sweating therapy is excellent for overall purification and balancing and can effectively be combined with other cleansing therapies. The skin is the largest eliminative organ in the body and the elimination through sweating is more passive and requires less expenditure of energy than elimination via the kidneys and bowels.

"The skin is the largest eliminative organ in the body."

Sweats were and still are practiced by many Native American people. Generally, a sweat-lodge is built around a circular hole which acts as a pit to hold glowing hot rocks. Water is then poured onto the hot rocks to provide a copious supply of steam. I have often participated in Native American sweat ceremonies and can attest to their effectiveness.

A number of years ago, I experienced a very intense traditional sweat led by a Native American man with amazing healing powers. During this sweat, a group of us sat around the firepit as a number of huge, glowing rocks were brought in on deer antlers. After the rocks were all in place, we began to chant and sing. Our leader made many prayers to help us through the difficult time of cleansing. The air was so hot and oxygen so scarce, that I could barely breathe. Negative feelings I didn't even know were in me began to come up. Our guide warned us about these feelings and said that it was our job to release them quickly and not hold on to them. We completed four 15-minute rounds of sweats—one for each of the cardinal directions (north, south, east, west). By the end of this process, I felt very limp and otherworldly. However, after a time I came back to myself, and then I felt an incredible lightness of spirit and body.

Now don't worry—it doesn't take a traditional sweat to gain the benefits of sweating therapy. A local sauna will do. Make sure you bring a sweating tea (equal parts yarrow, elder, and peppermint) and a willingness to let go of emotional and physical toxins. Usually three or four rounds of 15 minutes is sufficient. It is best to not overdo it the first time, especially if you are not used to saunas. Also, always get in cold water after the heat (a cold plunge is best). The colder the water the better, but don't stay in more than 30 seconds or a minute, depending on your constitution and how hot you are.

Caution: People with high blood pressure and heart disease, and people with weak constitutions or who are recovering from illness, should be careful in taking saunas. The heat can be debilitating if taken in excess, and plunging in water that is quite cold can affect the rhythm of the heart if it is prone to irregularity. Don't overdo the cold water. A short dip is usually all that is required.

Other Ways to Improve Elimination Through the Skin

Three other methods for improving elimination through the skin are the dry-brush skin massage, fresh-air bath, and a good old-fashioned hard physical workout.

Dry-Brush Massage: Using a good-quality natural bristle

brush, stimulate the skin all over the body. Start with small circular movements and progress to larger ones. The skin will become red, indicating that circulation and elimination are increasing. The brushing will usually loosen patches of dead skin, which can then be washed off. Removing this dead skin helps to increase the live skin's ability to absorb moisture and nutrients and to remove wastes.

Fresh-Air Bath: Whenever possible (and under conditions that Miss Manners would approve), remove all the clothes and bathe the entire body in fresh air and sunlight. Fresh air helps carry off harmful gasses and may provide important nutrients. Paul Bragg always stressed the importance of "Dr. Fresh Air." Unfortunately, modern clothing styles and/or materials often severely hamper the skin's access to fresh air.

Please note that it is best to not overdo exposure to the sun, especially if one is fair-skinned and blue-eyed and does not have a naturally dark skin. The planetary ozone layer, which protects us from harmful ultraviolet radiation, has been weakened to the point where cancer and other skin problems are on the rise.

Physical Exercise: There is nothing like a good physical workout for speeding elimination through the skin via the sweat. Whether it be hard work like chopping wood or digging holes, or more playful pursuits such as dancing, biking, or running, the result is the same: the increased respiration enhances elimination through the breath, extra muscle activity promotes lymph circulation, and of course sweating increases elimination through the skin.

Urinary Cleansing

The kidneys are another important avenue of elimination and should not be overlooked in the cleansing process. Many nitrogen-containing waste products, such as ammonia and urea, are excreted in urine. The liver transforms some fat-soluble toxins into water-soluble compounds that can be eliminated in urine. Some of the herbs that promote elimination through sweating, when drunk as a warm tea, will also promote elimination via the kidneys when used as a cool tea or tincture. To make a good urinary-cleansing tea, blend 1 part each of the following herbs.

Urinary-Cleansing Tea

Yarrow   Dandelion leaf
Elder flowers   Sarsaparilla
Cleavers

Directions: simmer 1 part of the herb blend in 5 parts of water for 10 minutes, adding 1 part peppermint at the end and steeping the herbs for about 10 minutes. Strain and store the tea in quart jars in the refrigerator. Drink 1/2 to 1 cup 2-3 times per day.

Intestinal and Bowel Cleansing

If we could see what accumulates in the colon over a period of 20 or 30 years, we would be appalled. It's not a pretty sight.

But, besides being ugly, waste accumulation has several unfortunate effects. First, it makes the exchange of nutrients and wastes between the inside of the bowel and the blood circulation less efficient. Second, it may interfere with beneficial bacteria or even harbor pathogenic (disease-promoting) bacteria. So from time to time, depending on the individual, one's diet, and other health considerations, it is good to do some kind of bowel cleansing.

In the old days, 50 years ago or more, the first thing to do for any disease was to take an enema. A few readers may remember their parents giving them a nice dose of castor oil at the first sign of a cold or tummy ache. I remember my mother telling me that

Table 21
Herbs for Intestinal and Bowel Cleansing

Herb	Action
Psyllium seed (powder)	high in soluble fiber; a good bulk laxative, and cleanser
Psyllium seed husk (powder)	very high in soluble fiber; excellent bulk laxative, cleanser
Apple or citrus pectin	very ionic; excellent for clearing heavy metals and environmental toxins
Burdock	stimulates the liver and gallbladder, increasing bile flow; high in inulin; cancer protector
Yellow dock	mildly laxative; stimulating to the liver and bowels
Fenugreek	cleansing and soothing
Flax	bulk laxative; high in essential fatty acids; reduces inflammation and irritation
Fennel	warming; removes gas; cleanses toxins; promotes and smoothes digestion

she and her sisters didn't dare get sick, because the consequence was often strong-tasting herb teas and castor oil. Although I don't believe that cleaning out the colon is the answer to all ills, a moderate amount of intestinal cleansing can be very helpful, especially for individuals who have had a Standard American Diet (SAD) for many years or who have consumed drugs or other harmful substances.

When doing an intestinal cleansing program, herbs can be a great help. Some of the better-known herbs for bowel cleansing are listed in Table 21. These can be used to make intestinal and bowel cleansing formulas that are taken orally. Substances such as pectin and clay, discussed below, also make good bowel cleansers and can be taken orally. A completely different strategy for cleansing the bowels and intestines involves the use of enemas and colonics. These latter methods are discussed in the following sections.

If you want to make your own colon cleanser, start with psyllium seed and husk, add herbs like yellow dock, burdock, dandelion, blessed thistle, or flax (in powdered form), then blend one teaspoon of this mixture into 6 to 8 ounces of water, and drink.

Important Note: Remember *always* to follow herbs high in soluble fiber (e.g., psyllium) with adequate water so as to keep the mass from getting stuck in the intestines and causing an obstruction. Two 6- or 8-ounce glasses of water or herb tea are usually sufficient.

If you prefer to leave the formulation of a bowel cleanser to the experts, there are many excellent commercial cleansing programs available in natural food stores. Many of them have detailed instructions included on the package or in accompanying small booklets.

Incidentally, besides being mildly laxative, soothing, and cleansing to the bowels, herbs rich in high-soluble fiber also have two other beneficial actions.   Laboratory and clinical studies show that they can help lower cholesterol (perhaps by limiting the uptake of certain fats), and they can help some people lose weight.

Clay and Pectin

Citrus or apple pectin, as well as bentonite clay, are excellent intestinal cleansers.   They are especially helpful in removing environmental toxins and radioactive substances from the body. Pectin is a large polysaccharide (sugar polymer), usually containing bound mineral ions like calcium and phosphorus. Apple and citrus peels are especially rich in pectin.   Pectin can also be purchased as a beige powder, which is then mixed as a tablespoon dose in water. Pectin powder will gel up in the body, drawing to it toxic chemicals because of its strong ionic (electrically charged) nature. Then breakdown products from the pectin will carry the toxins out of the body via the bowels. The old saying "an apple a day keeps the doctor away" may derive, in part, from the ability of the pectin in apple peels to cleanse the body. As a program, try the following:

1. Eat apples, organic bananas, pears, and other fruit in season for a few days, drinking at least 2 quarts of lemon-honey water per day. Make lemon-honey water by adding the juice of 1 lemon plus 1 tablespoon of honey to a quart of water and blending well.

2. Fast for the next three days, drinking mainly fresh apple juice, grapefruit juice, and lemon-honey water.

3. Start the fasting days with a pectin drink consisting of 1 tablespoon of apple or citrus pectin mixed in a glass of distilled water with a teaspoon of lemon juice. Follow with 2 cups of cleansing herbal tea, such as "Polari-Tea" or "Puri-Tea".

4. Take an enema every night, using a quart of lemon water.

Bentonite clay may be used instead of pectin in any cleansing program. Bentonite clay particles are extremely fine and, when ionized by sunlight, provide a powerful cleansing action. To use bentonite clay, mix 1 teaspoon of it in a glass of distilled water and stir well. Then set the glass in bright sunlight for about 6 hours, and drink. The sunlight helps ionize the clay particles. This gives them extra drawing power.

Enemas

The word *enema* is of Greek origin, and means simply to induce a bowel movement by injecting a liquid into the rectum. Enemas have been used for perhaps thousands of years as a means to remove noxious wastes from the colon and to relieve constipation or gas. An enema is not a very elegant procedure, but for those who need it, it can be quite effective and satisfying. Enemas can even be a life-saver for people who have a great deal of gas trapped in the colon which is creating sharp pain.

There has been some controversy in the past among health practitioners as to whether enemas should be used during periods of fasting or cleansing. My teacher, Paul Bragg, used to say that enemas were not often necessary and could even be habituating. In my experience, however, they can be useful during fasting and cleansing and are not habituating when used for short periods (not over one week). Used under these conditions, enemas can help the body remove waste products that may be thrown off into the bile, as well as putrefying material and bacteria generated in the colon itself. This may become especially important during a fast, when spontaneous bowel movements often cease. Then, by getting wastes out of the body with an enema, one can effectively keep reabsorption of these toxic substances to a minimum. Also, I think enemas may be more important today than they were 15 years ago, because of the many fat-soluble environmental toxins, such as pesticides and organic solvents, that have found their way into us through our drinking water, food, air, and other sources. Since many of these toxins circulate in the bile, it seems prudent to remove them from the body as quickly as possible.

Other situations where enemas may be necessary include:

- **For the elderly**, especially after long periods of inactivity, and/or when the colon has lost its tone due to overconsumption of highly processed foods;
- At any age after the **overuse of laxatives**, including stimulating herbal laxatives such as aloe and senna;
- When there is an uncomfortable buildup of **gas** in the colon, with resulting symptoms such as headache, general body aches, and even heart palpitations;
- When the **colon** is crippled by **inflammation**, overstretching, adhesions, and general weakening;
- For quickly **removing toxic materials** from the body. For instance, if one has ingested spoiled food, an enema can

remove more of the toxic material and bacteria than a regular bowel movement can and more quickly.

In case the reader is not familiar with the procedure for taking an enema, I will detail it here.

The best enema applicator is a fountain syringe. These are available at drug stores everywhere and are usually included with the standard rubber enema bags you can buy. A small, smooth applicator with a single end hole is also effective. A longer

Herbal Enema Teas

Here are several tea formulas to be used as enemas. For these teas, simmer roots, barks, and stems for 20 minutes, then let the tea cool for 10 minutes before straining and using it. Simmer leaves and flowers for 5 minutes, turn off the heat, then let the mixture steep for 10 minutes. A good starting proportion of herbs to water is 1:5, weight to volume. In other words, add one ounce of herb mixture to 5 ounces of water.

For gentle cleansing and mild liver stimulation:
burdock root, yellow dock, red clover, peppermint
1 part each

For mild cleansing and soothing action:

Dandelion root (35%)	*Licorice root (10%)*
Chicory root (30%)	*Marshmallow root (25%)*

For moderate cleansing and mild laxative effect:

Cascara bark (10%)	*Fennel (30%)*
Dandelion root (40%)	*Ginger (20%)*

For strong bowel cleansing and to dredge and cool:

Cascara bark (25%)	*Buckthorn bark (25%)*
Gentian (25%)	*Ginger (25%)*

Note: Start with only 1/2 cup of marked formulas per quart of warm water. Then adjust the amount for individual differences. Some people can easily take a full cup, others less.

applicator is not necessary. Be sure to lubricate the nozzle of the applicator with a little olive oil before use, and thoroughly sterilize the applicator after each use by boiling it or thoroughly cleansing it with soap and water.

The enema bag itself is placed at varying heights, depending on the desired results. If the liquid is meant to be retained in the colon for 10 to 20 minutes, it is best to hang the bag at a height of 2 or 3 feet above the level of the rectum. If more stimulation is desired and the liquid is to be expelled immediately, (the procedure recommended for removing gas), then the bag should be hung at 5 or 6 feet.

My usual practice is to start with 1 to 1 1/2 quarts of water heated nearly to body temperature. If the water is at room temperature or colder, it will often cause cramping soon after it is injected, which limits the time it can be retained. One can also add the juice of 1 lemon or 1 cup of herbal tea to the water. (See the sidebar on page 158 for appropriate herbal formulas.)

The two best postures for introducing the enema fluid into the colon are either lying on the back with the knees flexed (a pillow under the head adds to one's ability to relax), or on elbows (or chest) and knees with the rear end slightly raised.

After the fountain syringe or smooth tube is introduced, it is usually best to regulate the flow of fluid so that too much is not taken in at once. A very slow introduction of the fluid will cause less cramping and discomfort and will allow the fluid to reach a higher place in the colon.

Enemas can be repeated 2 or 3 times in succession, if necessary. To dissolve hardened fecal matter, warm water works best. It may take up to 5 or 6 treatments, each 20 minutes apart in order to loosen and expel the most encrusted matter.

Caution: If symptoms of dizziness, nausea, or light-headedness occur, it is best to stop the enema process. If you are not used to taking enemas, start slowly with only one application/day.

Special Therapeutic Enemas

Colitis. Add 1 quarter ounce of salt to 1 quart of water at a temperature of 105 to 115 degrees F. Then add 1 cup of tea made according to the formula below, and take the entire mixture as an enema. Note: Make sure to follow any salt enema with a pure water enema. It is not advisable to allow excess salt to remain in the colon.
   Chamomile (60%)
   Licorice (10%)
   Marshmallow root (30%)
Atonic or Severely Toxic Colon. A *cold water* enema is prescribed when the bowels are very weak and atonic, due to years of poor diet and lack of physical exercise. Cold water is used because it produces a very powerful stimulation, in the colon, thus strengthening the nerve force there and bringing tone to the bowel muscles. Also, when the colon is very toxic, a warm-water enema can actually dissolve toxins and make them more available for absorption through the intestinal wall. This can lead to unpleasant symptoms such as heart palpitations, nausea, and headache. If such a reaction should happen to you during a warm-water enema, follow it with a cold-water enema (of about 70 degrees F.), depending on your constitution.

For a cold enema, start with water at 85 degrees F., gradually reducing the temperature by 10 degrees in successive applications.

Eventually, a temperature of 50 degrees F. can be sustained.

Colonics

Colonics are simply deeper and more prolonged enemas. For the past 20 years, I have had a colonic or two every year. If the operator is skilled, one can feel that the cleansing of the colon is deeper with a colonic than with a simple enema. The procedure involves using a machine to fill the bowels with warm water. A return tube draws the water back out after 5 to 15 minutes. Usually two or three applications are given in one session.

Over the years, there has been some controversy about colonics. Critics say they are unnatural and therefore unnecessary. Proponents say that due to the modern refined diet, the body needs a little extra assistance in removing deeply encrusted fecal matter from time to time. My own opinion is that a program consisting of a 3-day fast with an enema every day, and finishing with a colonic or two, is a good thing.

Fasting

Throughout the ages, fasting has been used by spiritual leaders and health teachers. My introduction to the incredible benefits of fasting came from my teacher, Paul C. Bragg, life-extension specialist and author of many books on health, including *The Miracle of Fasting.* Paul Bragg, more than anyone, showed me how to fast, for how long, and how to break a fast in the right way.

In 1968, I was so sick and unhealthy from eating processed foods and junk food, and from overusing alcohol, various drugs, and coffee, that I was unable even to walk up a small hill without

Table 22
Benefits of Fasting

- **Saves Time**: Hours a day are often spent in working to pay for food, shopping, preparing food, eating, and cleaning up the kitchen.

- **Rest**: Give your digestive system a much-needed rest.

- **Increases Energy**: Tremendous amounts of vital energy usually spent in digestion, assimilation, and elimination are saved for other purposes, instead.

- **Spiritual Upliftment**: All great spiritual figures have fasted. Fasting helps cut our attachment to the physical world.

- **Cleansing**: The body is very wise. When it can't get energy from food, it breaks down diseased and second-rate or toxic cells, recycles the usable components, and eliminates wastes.

- **Lose Weight**: Not eating is one of the fastest ways to lose excess weight. Fat is broken down before muscle tissue in the fasting process.

- **Healing**: Even intractable diseases have been healed during fasts (see books on fasting in the Resource List, p. 291).

- **Breaks Addictions**: Fasting is one of the very best ways to break addictions. It can strengthen discrimination and will power. After a fast, the last thing you want to do is smoke a cigarette or drink coffee or alcohol. Many years ago, I broke my seemingly unbreakable addiction to tobacco with a fast.

- **Appreciation**: In no period of human history has such a variety of food been as readily available as today. There is so much abundance that it is easy to even become blasé about delicacies such as tropical fruits and artichoke hearts. Fasting helps us realize just how blessed we really are. I still vividly remember how delicious a bite of apple tasted after my first 2-week fast. The finest ambrosia of the Gods couldn't have been better!

getting strong heart palpitations and shortness of breath. I got to the point that I felt life was not worth living. Then one day I went into a natural foods store in Palm Springs, and looking at the books on display there, I noticed a copy of *The Miracle of Fasting*. I picked the book up and began leafing absent-mindedly through the pages. Something about the words written there hit home: the author seemed so enthusiastic and energetic, so sure that fasting and diet alone could alter the course of one's health and life.

Not being one to do things half way, I took the book home and began a fast, starting with an 8-ounce glass of raw broccoli juice. As you can imagine, I became quite ill. The next day I felt even worse—I ached all over as if I had a bad case of flu. I felt nauseous, dizzy, and very weak. But I stuck with a diet of mostly raw foods and especially juices and big salads, and miraculously, after about two weeks, I began to feel much better. Now, some 23 years later, I have tried about every diet system imaginable, and I have fasted many, many times. Based on my experience, there are a few key points to keep in mind in order to gain the maximum benefit from a fast.

Fasting Guidelines

1. Ease into and out of a period of fasting by eating fresh fruits and vegetables for two or three days. Never shock the body by changing from a heavy diet to fasting, or vice versa.

2. Speed up or slow down the cleansing process by selecting juices to suit your constitution, general state of health and cleanliness, the climate, and other factors. (see Table 23).

3. Do not continue a fast beyond 3 to 7 days, unless you

have plenty of experience fasting. If you have done at least a year of cleansing, you may fast for up to 2 weeks. Fasts longer than 2 weeks are used for special needs and require expert supervision.

4. How one breaks a fast is almost as important as the fast itself. Much of the good that is accomplished in a fast can be undone if the fast is broken improperly or if improper dietary habits are adopted or returned to after the fast.

The major benefits of fasting are listed and explained in Table 22 on p. 162. Below I will outline two effective fasting programs.

3-Day Juice Fast

For a novice faster, I usually recommend a short 3-day fast using fruit juices. Water fasts usually are too severe for most people and are probably not the best kind of fast for today's world of industrial chemicals and heavy metals that may be stored in our bodies. Besides, fruit juices contain pectin and other purifying substances that help remove toxic wastes.

Always eat raw fruits and vegetables for two or three days before and after the fast, to ease in and out of the fasting period. During the fast, drink nothing but water and freshly-extracted juices. If fresh juice is impossible to obtain during the fast, then use bottled organic grape or apple juice diluted in a 1:1 ratio with distilled water. However, even fresh-squeezed grapefruit juice and distilled water is preferable to bottled juices, because the body responds best to the vitality of fresh juice. Note that the whole process actually lasts 10 days counting preparation and transition to a normal diet.

My usual program for a 3-day fast is as follows:

Days 1-3 (Preparation): Upon rising, do 20-30 minutes of deep breathing and stretching (continue this throughout the fast). Then drink a liver flush as detailed on p. 145. Follow with two cups of cleansing tea. Eat raw fruits and vegetables, salads,

---

> *"When I complete the fast, I always emerge with a sharpened sense of discipline and greater faith in my own discrimination."*

---

whole apples, pears, grapefruit—but not bananas (juicy foods only). Drink as much distilled water with fresh lemon juice added to taste as desired. More herbal tea in the evening is optional.

Days 4-6 (The Fast): Start each day during the actual fast with the liver flush and tea, and follow one or two hours later with about 6-8 ounces of freshly-squeezed fruit juice (usually apple, grape, or grapefruit) diluted with distilled water in a 1:1 ratio. A few hours later, try 6-8 ounces of mixed vegetable juice, usually a combination of organic carrot and celery with a touch of beet or parsley. In the evening take another glass of fruit juice, and perhaps a cup of herb tea. Finally, before bed take an enema consisting of 1 quart of warm distilled water mixed with the juice of 1/2 lemon, as explained in the section on enemas on p. 156.

If you've never taken an enema before, you will be surprised at how much comes out. (Remember that during a fast the bowels will usually cease to move.) This will get out any waste material that is being eliminated into the colon and will also soften and remove old fecal matter that may be hanging onto the walls of the colon.

On the last day of the fast, I usually go to a professional for a colonic flush. This ensures that my colon is thoroughly cleaned. During the colonic, I am always amazed at what I see come out—even after fasting and taking enemas. Some people prefer to have a series of two or three colonics after a fast.

Day 7: I always break a 3-day fast with a raw salad, according to Bragg's instructions. I have tried different ways to break a short fast and have found this way the most satisfactory. The roughage in the salad helps move the bowels and acts as a sort of "broom" to sweep out further wastes. My first salad consists of grated cabbage, carrot, finely chopped celery, a little grated beet root, and perhaps some finely shredded romaine lettuce. I eat a good-sized bowl of this salad at about noon of the day after the 3-day fast (the 7th day overall). In the evening I eat more raw vegetables, or a little vegetable broth, depending on how I feel.

Day 8: Eat fruits and vegetables during the day, with the addition of a steamed potato or some steamed green vegetables.

Day 9: Begin to eat regularly, but lightly. Chew each bite well and combine foods carefully. I always find that by this time I desire no processed foods. It feels so good to have had the discipline and wisdom to fast that I don't want to put anything in my body that is not the very best fresh, organic food.

Suggestions:

I have never seen any serious problems during a fast, but it is common to experience symptoms such as:

√ dizziness

√ mild heart palpitations

√ weakness

√ light headedness

√ tiredness

√ forgetfulness

√ mild nausea

√ a bad taste in the mouth, known as "faster's breath"

√ a gnawing or empty feeling in the stomach and abdomen

If these become frightening or unpleasant, you can slow down the cleansing process by using a juice or broth that is less cleansing for a short time, until the symptoms abate. (See Table

---

Table 23
Cleansing Power of Fasting Liquids

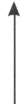

[MOST CLEANSING]
Water, distilled
Fruit juice, fresh-squeezed
Fruit juice, bottled
Vegetable juice, fresh-squeezed raw
Vegetable juice, bottled
Vegetable broth, cooked
Fruit, Fresh raw
Vegetables, fresh raw
Grains, cooked
Legumes, cooked
[LEAST CLEANSING]

23 for a ranking of relative cleansing strengths of various juices and broths.) Also, it always helps to rest, if possible, and to focus on the positive aspects of the cleansing and healing process. Envision the wastes leaving your body. I often imagine a pure mountain meadow filled with wildflowers and with a crystal clear stream flowing through it. I imagine myself bathing in the pristine water, and I think of all wastes leaving me and returning to mother earth, where they are broken down into pure elemental components.

During a fast you also begin to eliminate old drug residues and the "energetic field" of junk foods such as pizza and synthetic ice cream. When this happens, you may find that you develop an almost unbelievable craving for these things. It is during this time that I always ask for the grace and strength to get through the rough spots and continue on with the fast. If I feel as though I might succumb to these cravings, I read inspirational books such as *The Miracle of Fasting* in order to "psych" myself up on the whole process. Also, I always try to remember that I am not alone when I am fasting. Many people have fasted before me and have had the inner strength to go through their fears and negativity and come out healthier and purer. When I complete the fast, I always emerge with a sharpened sense of discipline and greater faith in my own discrimination. I realize even more that health is first and foremost built on two cornerstones—discipline and awareness.

Besides purely physical symptoms, many negative feelings about yourself and others may begin to surface during a fast. These are negative ancestral, karmic, and recent emotions that are being eliminated and briefly re-experienced. It is best to do positive affirmations during this time. Let these feelings go by like clouds across a blue sky. Know that they will pass. It is important to not get attached to anything that comes through.

Finally, don't be in a hurry to get back to a regular diet. We tend to overeat after a fast, because we sometimes feel somehow deprived. Focus instead on the tremendous cleansing you have just accomplished. Notice the increased clarity and efficiency of your bodily processes.

The 7-Day Fast

For the 7-day fast, simply follow the same general guidelines as for the 3-day fast. The same juices, broths, and teas can be used before, during, and after the fast: only the number of days you actually fast changes. After 3 days, the hunger will usually abate, which is a big help.

Contraindications for Fasting

- Fast with caution or avoid during pregnancy.

- Babies and young children should not fast or only under supervision.

- Caution after exposure to pesticides, herbicides, and other fat-soluble toxins.

- Avoid, do sparingly, or use kicharee fast (eat only mung beans and rice in soupy form) in deficiency conditions.

However, when doing a fast for longer than five days, one may experience alternating periods of strength and weakness or even dizziness and nausea. Unpleasant symptoms are especially likely if this is your first fast, or if you haven't fasted for awhile, or if you have had a diet high in junk foods, cooked oils, and animal protein. At night you may feel your heart beating more forcefully than usual, even becoming uncomfortable. This should be no concern, though. Try taking a relaxing herbal formula, such as the following one.

A 7-day fast should be broken more carefully than a 3- or 5-day fast. It is best to eat a small amount of fresh fruit, as this is the easiest to digest. Make sure to chew each bite for an extended period—really taste and enjoy that fruit! I often break a 7-day fast on two apples or an apple and some grapes. Don't overdo it, though; always eat less, if there is a doubt.

The second meal can be 3 to 4 hours later and can consist of

Relax Fast

Chamomile (1 part)
Passion flower (1 part)
Catnip (1 part)
Hops (1/2 part)
St. John's wort flowers (1/2 part) (or add 10 drops of the tincture to a cup of tea)
Optional: Linden flowers (1 part)
Honey (1/2 teaspoon per cup to taste)

more fruit or a small raw salad. The second day, start eating more raw fruits and vegetables. The third day, eat more of the same with the addition of some vegetable broth and lightly steamed vegetables. On the fourth day, you may eat more normally but still lightly and chewing carefully. Also, always watch food combining closely after a fast, as the digestive tract is not used to strange combinations, such as fruit and cooked protein foods. Gas will usually result if food combining is poor. It may take as much as a week after the fast for your digestion to return to its full capability. Nonetheless, your digestion should be more efficient and your appetite keen. You may experience energy rushes in various parts of the body, as well as a kind of exhilaration at times. If you ever feel achy and tired, this is often due to overeating or wrong food combining—in which case you should rest and eat more lightly for a meal or two.

Questions and Answers About Fasting

Q. Is it best to work or rest during a fast?
A. It is possible to work during a fast—in fact, at times you will feel as though you have boundless energy. Sometimes, however, you will feel weak or dizzy and will need to rest in a quiet place. I have often taken a "cleansing vacation" by fasting over a three-day holiday. What better way to spend one's vacation than resting the digestion as well as the mind and whole body? Remember that resting during a fast can make more energy available for cleansing and healing.

Q. How will I know when it is time to stop fasting?
A. It is best not to be too fixed about the number of days you fast. You may set out on a 3-day fast, and after 3 days feel so good and positive about the process that you decide to go on to 7 days. On the other hand, you may set out on a 7-day fast only to decide after 3 days that you have had enough. In that case you should break the fast. Also, remember that if unpleasant symptoms persist for more than a few hours, you can slow down the cleansing process by using the appropriate liquids.

Q. How often should I fast?
A Some people like to fast one day a week. I have done this for several months at a time and found it beneficial. Choose one day a week, such as Sunday, and make this a day of rest and physical regeneration in all ways. I feel that the very best time to fast is in the spring, as "spring cleaning."

This is a traditional ritual in many cultures. Many Native American peoples had their spring sweat lodges and vision quests, which included a period of fasting. In the Jewish faith, one often fasts during Yom Kippur. Bragg often recomended fasting in the spring and fall for 3 or 7 days each time. I have been doing this for a number of years.

Q. Will I feel hungry during the whole fast?
A. This varies from person to person, but I can say from experience that hunger often goes away after 3 days. That's one reason why people often want to continue on to 5 or 7 days after making it through the first 3 days, which are usually the hardest.

Q. Is fasting for everyone?
A. Obviously, each person has to decide for him or herself. I feel that fasting can be useful in many cases, especially in today's world of excess. However, it is important to note that fasting may not be appropriate for people who are "deficient" or weak. For instance, a fast may not be recommended for a person who, for a number of years, has been eating a cold "yin" diet consisting mainly of raw vegetables and fruit. On the other hand, though, fasting is especially good in "excess" conditions, where one has been eating a diet rich in meat and processed foods, or has been consuming drugs and alcohol on a regular basis. Thus, in summary, it is of vital importance that the individual constitution be taken into account.

Chapter 7

Types of Stress
and Stress-Reduction Techniques

As many of us are aware, excessive stress—or at least not dealing well with stress—has a negative effect on health in general, and especially on digestion. Some stress is necessary to stimulate growth as an organism, but when that stress becomes too much to assimilate, either because it is not the right kind of stress or is too prolonged, then problems will ensue.

Here we will consider three types of stress:

• **Ancestral stress** (usually from negative experiences during early childhood and family life)

• **Environmental stress** (from external sources, both physical and social)

• **Physical stress** (mechanical stress due to repeated or habitual use of the body in a certain way)

Ancestral Stress

In my experience, most of the stress we carry with us begins "from the beginning." It may go as far back as from some former time or existence or to some trauma in the womb. However, for most people the most immediate part of this stress derives from early dealings with parents and relatives. Ancestral stress is by far the hardest type of stress to deal with because it is so deeply ingrained in us. We can live next to a toxic dump site and have

174

crazy people for neighbors, but if we are whole, peaceful, balanced, and feeling good about ourselves, we can deal with the situation. It may not be easy, but we can deal with it. We would probably move somewhere else—however, even if we stayed, we could probably find some way to adapt and survive.

"So many digestive dysfunctions are directly caused by various ancestral stress factors."

On the other hand, if we are racked with ancestral stress and do not feel peaceful, balanced, and good about ourselves, no external environment, however perfect, can make us happy inside. We may have money, looks, brains, and doors opened for us by an influential family, yet still we will be miserable. No matter how much external grace we receive, we can't live up to the ideal our mother and father may have for us. Or they don't know how to express their love in a positive way and so we feel starved. Or we harbor resentments for our parents or others because we feel wronged or cheated. Or we have acquired such a bad self-image during our upbringing that no amount of success can erase it.

So many digestive dysfunctions are directly caused by various ancestral stress factors. We may "hold onto" our wastes and become constipated. We may feel inadequate and unworthy of love, so we don't allow ourselves to assimilate and utilize the

nutrients in our food. Or we may eat ravenously, even patho-
logically, to "insulate" ourselves from the world and from being
hurt by the lack of love we feel. But in the end, it always comes
down to an inability to share our own love with others, the sad
irony being that at heart all people have unfathomed depths of
love to share; we are an unending source of love.

To help us get "unstuck" and recover our innate health and
ability to love, many, many systems of therapy have been developed. A great number of these therapies are similar in that they
aim to help people become aware of and release negative family
patterns. One of the most effective methods I have found for
doing this is Gestalt Therapy, called "chairwork" by the people
who taught it to me at the Polarity Institute on Orchas Island,
Washington. In this type of therapy, negative family patterns are
explored and released through role-playing directed by a mediator
in front of an audience or group. You sit facing an empty chair
while the audience or group sits around you at a distance of
several feet, and the mediator sits to your side between your chair
and the empty one. Then you imagine someone sitting in the
empty chair, that is, someone you have something to say to, and
you start to speak to them as if they were really there.

For instance, you might put your boss in the chair and
express how angry you are with him or her: "You make me
sick!" "I hate your guts!" "You have the compassion of a hired
killer!" and so forth. Then the mediator draws you into a deep
dialogue with the imagined person. If the mediator is skilled,
you will eventually discover that no matter who you start with in
the opposite chair, and no matter how "right" you think you are,
you will usually end up talking to one or both your parents in the
other chair. Then suddenly you feel the sadness, emptiness,

loneliness, and futility of withholding your love and not accepting them for all they are. You will also learn that the very thing you are hating or yelling at in the "other" person is really right there inside you, and it is that presence in you and your attachment to it that is upsetting.

In my case, during this work I found I had some feelings for my mother that I was holding onto. She hadn't given me all the love and attention I thought I needed. Of course, there were many apparently unrelated scenarios and complicating relationships and plays in the way, but when it was all boiled down to its essence, this was the source of my pain. And I discovered, through the process of chairwork, that my mother was doing the best she could, based on what she received in the way of love and understanding when she was young. When I realized this, I was able to let the resentment go. I was able to appreciate and love her for what she did give, which was incredible. This released a tremendous amount of ancestral stress right there.

So how can you incorporate this technique into your life to explore and release ancestral stress? Working with a skilled mediator and a group of other people with whom you have formed a working bond is ideal. However, this situation is not always easy to find (for a list of centers that do this work, or variations thereof, see the Resource list on page 290).

Luckily, though, it is also possible to gain some benefit from role-playing by oneself. Simply sit opposite an empty chair with no one around and begin a conversation with someone you feel you need to say something to.

For instance, to use the example above, you might put your boss in the chair and say to her or him: "You make me sick. You don't even treat me like a human being." (Or say something less dramatic.) Then when the energy of your statement has blown over the empty chair, "switch" roles by going over and sitting in the other chair. The energy of your statement and emotions can be felt. If you play this honestly, you can really begin to get into the other role and feel how the other person feels. Playing the role of your boss, you might answer back, "Well, you are constantly making mistakes, and I can barely make ends meet in my business as it is. I can't afford to carry any dead weight"— or whatever else your boss would say. Surprisingly, we all know at some level what the other person really feels, and it only takes stepping aside from our "self" to acknowledge this.

"The only thing that is keeping us from this higher knowledge and perfection is ourselves."

Next, switch back and give your reply, e.g., "I do not constantly make mistakes. I made only that one last week, and I really try to do my work well, but you don't seem to notice." And continue in this manner back and forth. Eventually, you will see that the other person is not any different from you—he or she has the same need for love and appreciation and the same basic insecurities. When a deep realization of this fact comes, anger and separation melt. Then you can go on to work with people who have more meaning in your life such as your immediate family. And you will find basically the same things—that they need love, too, but they had or have a hard time expressing it, just as you may.

Again, if this type of therapy doesn't suit you, there are many others for exploring these ancestral patterns. In any case, the reason for this chapter, within the larger context of this work on digestion, is not to explain all the different techniques for working with ancestral stress, but to emphasize their importance. True healing cannot take place unless we work on these inner issues. Probably the real bottom line is that we have forgotten who we really are—we have a profound amnesia. We completely identify with all these patterns, concepts, and negative family attachments and fail to notice that the real being, the one who is timeless, radiant, and joyful is quietly there, always. The only thing that is keeping us from this higher knowledge and perfection is ourselves.

Environmental Stress

Environmental stress is of two types—physical and what might be called social or even better, socio-psychic. Stresses from the physical environment used to be easier to control and to adjust to than ancestral stress, but they are becoming increasingly less so. As individuals, we can recycle everything we use, use no processed foods or plastic packaging, walk everywhere and eschew automobiles as polluting beasts, and try to live in harmony with the earth—yet our planet becomes more polluted every day. In the future, this may pose challenges for adaptation. Luckily, though, even as our modern society goes against Nature, we still have Nature herself to protect us from our own folly and unawareness. Many natural medicines such as those discussed in this book can help us cope with and adapt to stresses from the physical environment.

Socio-psychic stress, however, is another sort of beast. This is the name I give to the stress caused by the collective force of people's thoughts and emotions, or energy fields. This type of "environmental problem" gets less press than the physical one, but that doesn't meant it's less real or less pernicious. If you've ever visited a very big city, you know what I mean. I go to a large metropolitan area usually twice a year, and over the years I have noticed a definite phenomenon. Within hours of landing in the city, I notice a dramatic change in my thoughts, feelings, and energy field. I feel a decided "lower chakra" effect. Any lofty thoughts or feelings I may have had before I arrived are replaced by feelings of restlessness, strange desires, and unsettling visions of fast cars, wild parties, and shopping sprees. Not that this is all that goes on in big cities—far from it. However, millions of people there do lead fast, fractured lifestyles, and their desires and thoughts are bound to create an energy field of immense proportions. Whether you want to think of the phenomenon as non-verbal expressions of social norms or psychic pollution, the net result is the same: the simple fact is that all the people around us influence us greatly. When this influence is negative, it is often difficult to keep centered and remain in a calm, balanced state.

Interestingly, socio-psychic stress can affect the physical body directly and usually manifests itself in the solar plexus or earth center—the area corresponding to digestion. When this happens, it is often good to "protect" the solar plexus by rubbing warm oils over the area. Pay special attention to any feelings of tenseness as well as to painful digestion. Take 10 or 15 minutes to massage these out, using circular strokes. Just being aware of the power of socio-psychic stress and bringing it to a conscious level is an important step in counteracting its harmful effects on digestion.

Physical Stress

What I mean by physical stress is actual mechanical stress— excessive work stress placed on part of the body, causing that part to wear out prematurely. For instance, if you are an editor who constantly reads during work, as well as using your eyes for normal daily activities such as reading for pleasure or watching television, then over time your eyes will probably wear out faster than if your hobby were tennis, running, or other sports activities. Similarly, if you are very sports-minded and not only enjoy running, playing tennis, swimming, and biking for pleasure, but also play tennis for a living, then you may wear out your elbows or knees fairly quickly.

This concept of wear and tear was crystallized for me by an article in *National Geographic* about the great Russian writer, Tolstoy. Each day, he consciously changed his activity several times, in order to exercise different parts of his body and mind and to keep active and in shape. For instance, since he was a writer, he began his day by writing for several hours. Then he would do some heavy physical work, such as building or gardening. Following this, he would do some kind of craft-work with his hands, such as building a birdhouse. At the end of the day, he would take time to socialize with his friends, simply relaxing in a congenial atmosphere and laughing and exchanging ideas. Thus, every part of his being was exercised but not overworked.

Now a balanced lifestyle (Tolstoy's being the ideal example) helps create strong and steady digestion. Being a writer and scholar myself, I have developed the mental side of my being extensively. Fortunately, I have been an active person most of my life and have enjoyed being outside, observing nature, and looking at flowers. This has saved me from excessive physical stress up until the last few years, when I have become more and more involved with my research and writing. Today, although I tremendously enjoy my work, at times the long hours of sitting and concentrating make my digestion less efficient than usual. I have found that during times of intense mental work—a type of work more and more people do today in their jobs in this new "information age"—it is especially important to take a "digestive break" and move the energy that has been channelled up to the mind back down into the body. Have you ever noticed that after lunch you have difficulty concentrating on work? This is partly due to an initial blood sugar drop subsequent to eating and partly to energy being directed to digestion rather than mental processes.

"The best way to release physical stress or tension is by exercising."

So how does one control or minimize physical stress? For one, I have found that eating many small meals throughout the day, rather than a couple of big ones, helps keep my blood sugar and my energy constant. However, the best way to release physical stress or tension is by exercising. In fact, I would place exercise or sports at the top of the list for techniques to deal with emotional and mental stress as well.

A word about exercise: Although there are as many ways to move the body as there are people, some types of exercise are less stressful on the body than others, and some are more suitable for individuals with certain types of constitutions than others. Below are some comments on a number of popular exercises that I have found to benefit digestion and general health. Remember, too, that much of the energy that could be directed to keep the functions of assimilation and elimination at top efficiency, is often directed needlessly to the muscles. For instance, when the sympathetic nervous system is activated by taking stimulants such as coffee, tea, chocolate, or cola drinks, it sends energy to the muscles for a "flight or fight" reaction. If you engage in sports, this muscular energy can be discharged. However, if all you do is sit at a desk, then the energy becomes stagnant and congeals in the muscles, creating soreness and tension.

Exercises to Reduce Stress

Walking: Walking may be the best form of exercise for the digestion. It is not an intensely aerobic sport, and it does not place a great stress on any part of the body. I consider walking one of the best health tonics available, at any price—and it is usually free! Recent research shows that walking can be as effective as more vigorous activities, such as running, in protecting the heart and blood vessels against disease, reducing weight, and releasing stress.

The big question for walking is where to walk? If you live in the middle of a big city like New York, finding a healthful place to walk may be something of a challenge. Still, there are beautiful parks in nearly every city. When walking, it is best to let go of all the tensions created in the mind. Try not to think about anything in particular—be a watcher instead. Watch the children, flowers, trees, cars, people, dogs, whatever. And experience the world fully with your senses. Bring full consciousness into your body—your legs, feet, arms, fingers, and especially the abdomen. Also, imagine the digestive organs working at their maximum efficiency. If your mind wanders to problems, comparisons, and so forth (as it will), bring it back again and again to the state of watching. Try to energize the doer and the watcher, instead of noticing that you are thinking or comparing. Just watch everything and don't judge it or make a quality out of it. Apprehend everything with your whole being.

If you walk in this fashion, you will free up tremendous amounts of energy for the digestive process, for when energy is released from mental work or fretting over attachments, it automatically flows to where it is needed most. Thus, if your digestion has been chronically weak, then energy will go to the digestive organs and help restore and regulate their functions. If you do not have enough energy to walk far, try at least to get up and slowly walk five minutes each day. Remember to inhale deeply, hold it for a few seconds, and then exhale fully. (Deep breathing is essential to digestion and the proper utilization of energy throughout the body.) Build up the time spent in walking each day by adding five minutes each week to your routine, until you are walking 30 minutes in the morning and 30 minutes in the evening, after dinner. Although vigorous activity after meals is not good because it diverts energy from the digestive organs to the muscles, light activity is actually beneficial, because it helps move the blood and lymph and helps us to relax. Walking, especially, I have found, helps to promote assimilation of nutrients and elimination of wastes.

Running: Running or jogging is beneficial for all processes of the body, provided you run correctly. It is best to run on a soft surface, such as sand, a dirt or short-clipped grass track, or a path through a forest. Running on pavement is hard on the knees and shocks the body generally. Such stress is fine for occasional runs, but if repeated frequently, it can chronically weaken various parts of the body.

Running improves circulation and consequently the exchange of nutrients and wastes in all the tissues and organs of the body. This greatly enhances the digestive function.

Dancing: Dancing has all the advantages of running, plus more. Dancing can give you an aerobic workout, plus it allows you to express your creative energy to the fullest extent. Dancing also increases flexibility, and it is something you can do with others. Thus, it provides a great deal of nourishment on many levels. I have been an avid dancer for years and have found that a few hours of vigorous dancing can remove digestive stagnation and help release static energy stored in the muscles and emotional body.

Singing: Singing, like dancing, helps express and energize your creative side, and it is excellent for letting go of unexpressed feelings. Feelings, such as anger or grief, tend to be dissipated well by sounds. Singing also exercises and stretches the diaphragm (the large, dome-shaped muscle that separates the lungs from the stomach and digestive cavity). When this muscle is tight, as it often is after years of stress or unexpressed emotion, breathing

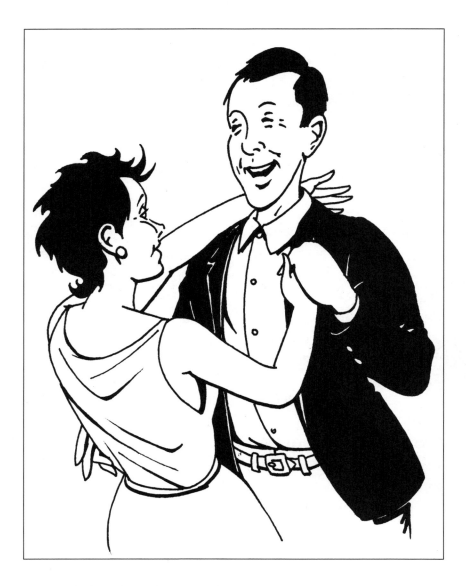

is impeded and pressure on the stomach and liver can constrict these organs, reducing their working capacity. In fact, singing is one of the best exercises for stretching and loosening the diaphragm. When singing, try to draw the air down into the abdomen as you inhale, allowing this area to expand. Then let the air come up into the chest to vocalize. This type of breathing is called *breath support*. With practice and proper breath support, you will find that you can develop increased vocal range and control, and a richer tone. I recommend that you sing at least two times a week for two hours. You can sing alone—though singing with others might be more enjoyable.

"Being in nature among the trees and wild plants is soothing and rejuvenating to the body and soul."

Swimming: Swimming is one of the best all-around exercises because it is aerobic, yet it does not stress the feet and knees. Swimming also stretches and strengthens the lower and upper parts of the body, while the stimulation of the cold water tonifies the circulation, digestion, and nerves. In other words, swimming has it all.

Weight-training: Weight-training has many advantages for overall health when practiced properly. It tones and relaxes energy from the muscles, makes doing physical tasks easier, and can improve one's self-image. It is also aerobic when practiced properly and can improve cardiovascular fitness. I have found that more repetitions with smaller weights generally provide excellent exercise and reduce the possibility of injury or strain.

Weight-training should not be attempted for at least an hour or two after eating a large meal and probably not for an hour after a small meal, because the strain it produces on the body and cardiovascular system diverts large supplies of energy from the digestion. Also note that, in some people, weight-training can over-activate the sympathetic nervous system, which increases overall tension.

Weight-training may also be contraindicated for people who have chronic adrenal weakness due to years of stress or overwork (kidney yin or kidney Qi deficiency in TCM). In this case, it should be practiced slowly with light weights until the adrenal weakness is on the way to recovery.

Biking: Bicycling is another exercise that helps release energy from the muscles, is aerobic, and increases oxygenation of the tissues. Because of the constantly changing scene, unlike running, bicycling can distract the mind and provide good mental release. The pumping of the legs and thighs massages and stimulates digestive organs and is one of the best ways I know to relieve chronic bowel tension. Indeed, because of this motion, bicycling can even relieve irritable bowel syndrome in some people (especially if due to pent-up nervous or emotional energy). It is important to warm up before biking very far or up steep hills; otherwise, the lower back and legs can be strained or even injured. Always work up to longer rides by doing short ones for a few weeks first, depending on your level of muscle tone and fitness.

Hiking: Back-packing or hiking in wilderness areas is one of the best therapeutic activities available—and again, it is usually free. Being in nature among the trees and wild plants is soothing and rejuvenating to the body and soul. After hiking with a heavy pack (remember to work up to it), it is amazing what one can digest!   I have often literally felt food dissolving and recombining in my body to form strong, healthy muscles and heat.   Sweating and increased urination and bowel movements are other excellent benefits of vigorous hiking.

Surfing: Surfing is an excellent sport for many of the reasons swimming is—the vigorous motion and the cold water.   However, if you surf mostly in cold water, be forewarned that continuous exposure to cold water tends to chill and weakens the kidneys. Also, the fear you may sometimes feel when staring at a 30-foot wave coming right at you can harm the kidneys and liver.   For these reasons, it is best to wear a wet-suit or special belt over the kidney area (a kidney warmer) to help protect these organs, as appropriate for your climate and constitution.

Skiing: Cross-country skiing can be exhilarating and aerobic. It provides solitude, stretches both the lower and upper body, and the cold, fresh air is certainly invigorating.   One only has to watch the fear factor, which shuts down the kidneys, liver, and bowels.   After skiing, it is important to relax for half an hour before eating a meal of any size.

Yoga: Yoga is an ancient Indian philosophy and way of being. Although one often thinks only of the physical exercises, or postures, of yoga, the full Indian concept of yoga entails integrating body, mind, and spirit in all areas of one's life.   For stress relief, the physical exercises alone can be of great value, but adding daily meditation and breathing exercises is much better. There are a number of excellent books available on the living art of yoga, as well as video tapes.

Tai Chi: Tai Chi is an ancient Chinese form of active physical meditation.   Through physical movement, one's mind and body is harmonized. As one progresses, the movements become more profound attuning one to larger cycles of the seasons and the phases of one's life. Although Tai Chi is a very meditative, gentle form of exercise, it can bring great strength and balance. There are several types of Tai Chi, some of which are more vigorous and emphasize physical strength. As in Yoga and the ancient Chinese practice, Qi Gong, breath is an integral part of the exercises.

Chapter 8

Programs for Common Digestion-Related Complaints

1. Poor Digestion Due to Congested or Overworked Liver

Diagnostic symptoms: Soreness in the liver area under moderate fingertip pressure; painful digestion; gas pains; constipation (less than 1 bowel movement per day); feeling of fullness in stomach and intestines; loss of appetite; PMS; depression; marked distaste for oily foods.

Dietary recommendations: Rest the digestive tract and liver by allowing at least 12 hours between the evening and morning meals. After seven at night, eat only small portions of fruit or drink herb tea. Exercise or do some physical work in the morning before eating breakfast. A moderate walk after a large meal will help stimulate the digestive juices. Do not overeat. Try skipping a meal (lunch), and eat light, easily digested foods such as steamed vegetables and raw salad greens (make some of these bitter). Eat semi-sweet fruits such as apples and pears in moderation. Add olive oil to food in teaspoonful doses, and go easy on cooked or refined oils.

Do the liver flush (see instructions in Chapter 6) for 1 week on, 2 days off, and 1 week on. This cycle can be repeated for 1 month but not more than 2 months. Enemas are of some benefit when there is a history of heavy, refined foods in the diet.

191

Herbal recommendations: Take herbs that decongest the liver, increase blood flow, and have an opening, slightly warming action. I recommend the following basic formula:

Liver Decongestant Tea

Dandelion root (1 part)   Burdock root (1 part)
Mugwort (1/4 part)   Ginger (1/2 part)
Fennel (1/2 part)   Milk thistle extract (1 capsule)

Directions: This formula can be mixed together in powdered form and encapsulated. Take 2 capsules 3 times per day. The formula can also be taken as a tea, in which case you should mix 1 ounce of whole herbs with 5 pints of water. Simmer (decoct) for 20 minutes, remove from heat, and let stand for 10 minutes before bottling or drinking. Drink 1/4 to 1/2 cup of warm tea 3 times per day. For convenience, make 1 quart of tea at a time (keeping relative proportions of herbs the same), and store in refrigerator. Always warm up the tea before drinking it. Note: the mugwort is optional, where available.

Remember, this is a strong medicinal blend and as with all such formulas, it is best to start with small doses—perhaps only several tablespoons per dose at first. Then work up to the full recommended dose after a few days, being sure to check for individual sensitivities and reactions as you go. Note that if your condition is mild, this tea is not for you; drink "Polari-Tea" or "Puri-Tea" instead (see section on Liver Flushes in Chapter 6). Both of these are milder and taste better and can be taken several times a day, as desired.

Incidentally, if you want to kick the coffee habit, you can brew a nice cup of coffee-substitute using roasted chicory and dandelion (add a kitchen spice or two, such as ginger, cardamon, or fennel, for warming action and flavor enhancement).

Other Recommendations: Massage the liver area by lying flat on your back and pressing your fingertips up under the right side of your ribcage. Use increasingly deep, circular motions, until all soreness or tightness is relieved (if soreness persists for more than a week, or if there is a pronounced tenderness in the area, it may be wise to seek the aid of a skilled natural health practitioner). Too much sitting and too little physical activity can block up the intestinal and liver area. It is good to massage this area often and to eat lightly until this condition improves.

I have also found from experience that one of the most harmful influences on the liver and digestion is excessive thinking. Sitting and staring at a computer monitor all day is especially nefarious. Two of my greatest allies in balancing my own life in this regard are walking and meditation.

2. Poor Fat Digestion

Diagnostic symptoms: Feeling of nausea or soreness in gut after fatty meals; burping with an oily taste in the mouth or throat; avoidance of or revulsion to fatty foods.

Dietary recommendations: Rest the digestive tract and take liver flushes, as explained in the section on congested liver, above. One of the best and most obvious remedies is to avoid foods cooked or fried in oil.

Herbal recommendations: Take herbs to increase bile flow,

> ## Milk Thistle/Artichoke Tea
>
> *Milk thistle seed extract (1 part)*
> *(1 dropperful or 1 tablet*
> *of the extract per cup)*
> *Artichoke leaves (1 part)*
> *Dandelion root (1 part)*
> *Mugwort (1/4 part)*
> *Yellow dock root (1/2 part)*
> *Peppermint leaf (1/2 part)*
> *Sweeten to taste with stevia herb*
>
> **Directions:** Warm the tea to room temperature and drink 1/4 to 1/2 cup of the tea before meals, especially fatty meals.

especially the above milk thistle/artichoke combination.

Other Recommendations: If nausea after fatty meals persists, it might be an indication of a deep-seated liver imbalance, in which case I recommend seeking the help of a skilled natural health practitioner.

3. Irritable Bowel Syndrome

Diagnostic symptoms: Burning or uncomfortable feelings in the bowels; alternating diarrhea and constipation; frequent gas and rumbling sounds in the intestines. These symptoms are usually worse after stress or when tired. There may be periods that are symptom-free, then times of pronounced symptoms.

Bowel diseases or imbalances are extremely difficult to diagnose. Pains can move from one area of the abdomen to another. Other possible ailments showing similar symptoms include appendicitis, diverticulitis, microflora imbalance due to antibiotics or other chemical factors, gallstones, and even cancer. However, always remember that cancer is the least likely. Nonetheless, it is wise to consult a qualified health practitioner if symptoms are serious enough or go on for more than a week or 10 days.

Dietary recommendations: Feed the beneficial flora in your intestines with foods containing ample soluble and insoluble fiber. Such foods include lightly cooked apples and other fruits, steamed vegetables, and grains that are easy to digest and are usually non-allergenic (i.e., millet, buckwheat, corn, and especially rice). Half-refined white rice is easier to digest than brown rice. Do not overeat or eat complex combinations—keep things simple. Sometimes several smaller meals during the day are easier to

Herbal Slime Tea

Flax seed (1 part)   *Fenugreek (1 part)*
Marshmallow root (1 part)   *Caraway seed (or Fennel)*
Licorice root (1/4 part)   *(1/4 part)*

Directions: Simmer the ingredients in water for 40 minutes, then remove from heat and allow to steep for 15 minutes. Strain the tea and store it in the refrigerator in quart jars or other suitable containers. The tea can be used for up to 5 days, if kept cool. Drink the tea as often as possible. I carry my teas with me wherever I go, sipping them or drinking a cup every hour or two.

handle than one or two big ones. Also, eat most foods lightly to well-cooked, and avoid common allergenic foods such as wheat, dairy products (especially pasteurized dairy), and eggs.

Herbal recommendations: I have had excellent results using the high-mucilage tea on the previous page.

Other Recommendations: Be sure to follow the programs for promoting beneficial microflora recommended in Chapter 4. It is essential to maintain a healthy microflora in any kind of bowel ailment. Research is increasingly identifying disordered microflora as a cause or contributing factor in irritable bowel syndrome and related bowel imbalances.

4. Gas (Flatulence)

Diagnostic symptoms: A bloated feeling accompanied by various pains in the abdomen or side; frequent passing of gas. Gas pains usually come and go and are not exercise-related. In fact they may be relieved by movement. Applying pressure with the fingers to different abdominal areas will usually aggravate the pains. Note that gas pains can radiate into the lower chest cavity, mimicking a heart attack. If these symptoms persist, consult a qualified health practitioner.

Dietary recommendations: Keep food combinations simple. Sugars mixed with protein foods will often lead to gas. Soak legumes for one or two days before cooking. Pour off the soak water a few times and refill with fresh water. Be sure to cook beans for at least 1 hour. Note that some people cannot tolerate certain legumes, such as garbanzos or lentils, well. If so, then these will consistently produce gas. (Bowel bacteria break down sugars called *trisaccharides* that are not well-absorbed in the small intestine.)   Also, avoid allergenic foods, especially pasteurized milk products.   Gas is a common symptom of lactose intolerance.

Herbal recommendations: Carry a small vial of peppermint oil with you at all times.   Whenever you need to, place 2 or 3 drops of this oil in a cup of hot tea or hot water, stir well, and drink.   Peppermint tea is also helpful, but not as strong as the oil. The following blend of traditional *carminative* or gas-relieving herbs is also helpful as a tea.

Other Recommendations: Again, see Chapter 4 regarding intestinal microflora.   Beneficial bacteria should be taken consistently.   Take at least 10 billion organisms per day if symptoms are severe, or 3 to 6 million if less severe.   Certain stretching or yoga postures can help relieve gas.   Lie on the floor face-down, put your arms under your head and your rear end up in the air.   Also, try massaging the abdominal area in circular, clockwise motions. Or, take an enema, one of the quickest remedies for gas known. The vacuum created as the enema water is expelled can literally suck out any gas caught in the bowels.

Pass on Gas Tea

Peppermint (1 part)   Fennel (1/2 part)
Ginger (1/2 part)   Cardamon (1/4 part)
Lemon peel (1/4 part)   Licorice (1/4 part)

Directions: Simmer the herbs for 20 minutes, let the blend steep for 10 minutes (unless you can't wait!), and drink as needed. Two drops of peppermint oil/cup of tea can be added for extra effect.

5. Skin Disorders (Acne, Psoriasis)

Diagnostic symptoms: Appearance of acne or psoriasis. Skin is irritated, red, oily, itchy, and inflamed. Bowel movements may have a strong, unpleasant odor.

Dietary recommendations: Although mainstream dermatologists generally do not consider diet to play a role in acne, I can assure you that this is not the case. I suffered from acne for many years when I was younger, and I learned by trial, error, and education what did and did not work. Since then, I have used natural remedies with many people to help alleviate this problem. I have found that, as far as food goes, it is important to make about 70 to 80% of the diet whole, natural, unprocessed foods. Focus on steamed and raw vegetables, whole grains and legumes, and fish or chicken (if desired.) Strictly avoid processed foods with a high oil content, such as candy bars, chips, ice cream, and pizza. Be moderate with dairy products—eat only small amounts of cheese; use olive oil instead of butter; and avoid pasteurized cow's milk. If you do nothing else but follow this diet, I can almost guarantee results within a month or so.

Herbal recommendations: Take cool and cleansing herbs. I like dandelion, burdock root, and burdock seed as liver/skin cleansers. Oregon grape root is a classic for skin conditions in general. Milk thistle seed extract is the most remarkable herb for psoriasis. One doctor I know who has used this extract in treating psoriasis has found that at least 50% of his clients improve both clinically and subjectively. Milk thistle has been used widely in Europe, proving highly effective in protecting the liver from environmental toxins and excess free radicals (see my booklet, *Milk Thistle, the Liver Herb,* for more information). Milk thistle

Skin-Cleanser Tea

Burdock root (1 part)   *Oregon grape root (1 part)*
Burdock seed (1/2 part)   *Dandelion root (1/2 part)*
Licorice (1/4 part)
(Fennel seed can be added for flavor)

also works inside the liver cells to increase the production of proteins and enzymes, thus helping damaged tissues to rebuild themselves. It is a most amazing herb, and I highly recommend it. I also recommend the following tea as a general skin cleanser:

Other recommendations: Apply hot and cold hydrotherapy to affected parts. First use hot compresses, or simply splash the face repeatedly with hot water, until a good flush occurs. Then repeat the process with cold water, though with about half the number of splashes. Hydrotherapy brings fresh blood to the affected skin, stimulating a general increase of deep circulation in the area. Ideally, you should repeat this procedure several times a day. However, if that is not possible, do it at least first thing in the morning and just before retiring at night.

Hydrotherapy will also remove excess oil and dirt particles from the skin, making the use of commercial soaps unnecessary. Soap disrupts the natural protective coating of fatty acids and microflora on the skin, thus inviting pathogenic bacteria to set up camp. I have not used soap on my skin for over 15 years (except on my hands to remove grease and stubborn dirt). In that time, hydrotherapy has made my skin healthier and clearer than before. I have also seen many other cases in which these two factors—improved circulation and proper cleansing—have eliminated chronic acne. Make sure to review the programs in Chapter 4, as probiotic therapy can be of great help.

6. Emotional Imbalances

Diagnostic symptoms: Excessive or lingering anger, sadness, or depression.

Dietary recommendations: Keep the liver open and clear by using the liver flushes described in Chapter 6, walking and deep breathing, and the dietary recommendations outlined in Chapter 3. Overeating is common in excessive emotional states, which only compounds the problem by further overloading the liver. The remedy is to eat lightly and to eat more fresh fruits and vegetables.

Herbal recommendations: I recommend the following herbal tea:

Emotion Ally-Tea

Dandelion root (1 part)	*Ginkgo leaf (1 part)*
Milk thistle seed tincture	*Lavender (1/2 part)*
(1 dropperful)	*Ginger (1/2 part)*
Damiana (1/2 part)	*St. John's wort (1/2 part)*

Sweeten with stevia herb or a little licorice. Avoid concentrated sweeteners like honey, because they can aggravate emotional swings.

Other recommendations: Try to release "stuck" emotions in constructive ways, such as heavy exercise or physical work. Crying and laughing, as long as they are not excessive, are helpful. Aromatherapy (the use of herbal scents) is also valuable in balancing emotional states. Try smelling lavender oil every so often during the day to brighten your spirits. I often carry a fresh flowering top of lavender in my pocket to sniff when I feel the need. Bach flower remedies work particularly well with emotional states. I recommend seeking out a Bach flower practitioner when dealing with long-term emotional imbalances.

7. Overweight, Obesity

Diagnostic symptoms: Sluggish metabolism; perhaps low energy.

Dietary recommendations: A diet of fresh fruits and vegetables, whole grains, and legumes is often the best. Keep oils to an absolute minimum, as well as meat, dairy, nuts, and eggs. These are highly concentrated foods that usually need to be eaten only in small amounts. This diet can be supplemented with lean fish such as sole, snapper, and halibut, if desired. The "bottom line" (no pun intended) for diet: keep it whole and fat-free.

Herbal recommendations: If excess weight is due to sluggish metabolism, (perhaps an underactive thyroid), the herbs bladderwrack (in capsule or tea form), and/or the East Indian herb guggul may be helpful. These have been recommended by herbalists to support proper thyroid activity. Cayenne in capsules (2 capsules 3x daily) may also be helpful as a general metabolic stimulant. This will actually "turn up" the metabolism.

A general bowel cleansing program or fasting program can

Weightless Tea

Bladderwrack (1 part)   *Chickweed (1 part)*
Burdock root (1/4 part)   *Alfalfa (1/4 part)*
Ginger (1/4 part)   *Licorice root (1/4 part)*

also be of great benefit. Try the above tea blend.

Other Recommendations: Proper exercise, especially dancing, swimming, bicycling, and lots of walking, is necessary and healthful in every way. Of course, don't overdo it. Start slowly if you are not used to exercising and work up to 20 minutes every other day. An hour of physical exercise or more every day is ideal.

8. Hepatitis or Cirrhosis (Liver Fire or Heat in TCM)

Please note: Hepatitis and cirrhosis are serious diseases that require the attention of a qualified health practitioner.

Diagnostic symptoms: Cirrhosis is a chronic, pathological inflammation of the liver, usually resulting in scarring and loss of liver function. In extreme forms it is potentially lethal. Cirrhosis can be caused by chronic hepatitis or alcohol and drug abuse. Symptoms for hepatitis and/or cirrhosis include headaches; facial flushing; red and inflamed gums; tenderness in liver area; diarrhea or loose, watery stools; yellow coating on the sides of the tongue. Often one experiences a profound fatigue and loss of a feeling of well-being, or migraine headaches.

Dietary recommendations: First of all, remove the stress factors that are creating the inflammation in the first place, whether they be excessive alcohol, drugs, or fried, spicy, and heavy foods (such as large quantities of red meat). Note that some cases of hepatitis are caused by an auto-immune disorder in which the body's own immune system attacks the liver. If this is the case, try a regimen of ginkgo leaf extract (24%)—2 or 3 40 mg tablets per day—and a few months of deep immune-strengthening herbs such as astragalus, ligustrum, codonopsis, shiitake, and reishi (take these as a tea or buy a commercial preparation). However, please note that it is difficult to differentiate between auto-immune and other types of hepatitis. For this reason, if the symptoms seem to worsen, or if no benefit is seen with the immune herbs, discontinue taking them. Again, with a serious disease such as hepatitis, it is always advised that you work directly with a qualified health practitioner.

A light diet built on greens, grains, and legumes is the best. Don't eat too many raw foods—take them lightly steamed instead. "Superfoods" rich in micro-nutrients and high-quality proteins are essential. These include steamed nettles, spirulina or other blue-green algae, and whole almonds (if your digestion is weak, soak the nuts in water overnight). Walnuts, too, contain valuable proteins and omega-3 fatty acids that can help decrease inflammation in the body. Keep the eliminative channels open by drinking plenty of pure water. Avoid spicy, warming foods such as garlic, cayenne, hot peppers, and curries. Let food cool to almost room temperature before eating. Also, as usual, don't cook foods in fat or oil for awhile—steam them instead.

Herbal recommendations: The major herb for hepatitis and cirrhosis is milk thistle (*Silybum marianum*). Take it as a tablet in concentrated, powdered, extract form. An average therapeutic dose of the 75% or 80% standardized extract is 1 tablet 3 or 4 times daily. A 10% standardized extract is also available, often blended with other liver-protective and healing herbs such as turmeric, artichoke leaf, gentian, and ginger. Of this latter preparation, take 1 or 2 tablets 3 times daily.

Try the following herb formula as a tea. Drink 1 to 3 cups per day, if it seems helpful.

Hepato Tea

Dandelion root (raw or dried, not roasted) (1 part)

Oregon grape root (1/2 part)

Turmeric (1/4 part)

Gentian root (1/8 part)

Artichoke leaves (1 part)

Licorice (1/4 part)

Ginger (fresh) (1/8 part)

Other Recommendations: Moderate walking and deep breathing are helpful. Antioxidant herbs, such as rosemary, hawthorn, and ginkgo, can be taken in addition to the above formula if the liver heat derives from heavy processing of toxins.

9. Drug Addictions (with accompanying liver stress)

Diagnostic symptoms: In addiction, even after one stops using the drug, usually some of the addictive substance remains circulating in the body for a time. This perpetuates the craving for it, which makes kicking habits a challenge—as I'm sure many readers know. Both nicotine and THC (the active principle in marijuana), for instance, remain in the body long after one quits smoking. The thing to do, then, is to eliminate all traces of old drugs from the body, and this often takes a few weeks or even months of cleansing.

Dietary recommendations: The liver flush is ideal for removing drug-related toxins from the body. Add to this fasting with fresh vegetable and fruit juices as a means to quickly eliminate addictive substances. Fast for three to five days at a time, eating mostly steamed and raw vegetables afterwards. For extra cleansing, eat only fruits between fasts. Some sweating and lots of fresh water and oxygen (deep breathing and vigorous exercise) will also help with the process of elimination.

Herbal recommendations: See my formula on the following page for eliminating addictions. I call it "The Tea-Totaler."

A word about golden seal: I have been asked about using it to pass drug detection tests so many times that I've lost count. It has become a fad to use golden seal for this, and thousands of bottles of the herb are apparently being sold in health food stores all over the country. However, according to the research that Foster (1989) did on the subject, there is no clinical or laboratory basis for this use. My own theory on the matter is that beyond any placebo effect golden seal might have (I have had people tell me that it worked for them), it might have an overall cleansing effect on the liver, thus enhancing the body's eliminative process. If this is so, then the above tea and other recommendations in this section would certainly be more effective than pure golden seal. Also, I must warn you that golden seal is potentially toxic if taken for more than 10-14 days in large amounts.

"Tea-Totaler" Tea

Dandelion root (1 part)   Wild oats (1 part)

Milk thistle tincture or extract   Passion flower (1/2 part)

   (about 1 dropperful,   Lobelia (if obtainable)

   40 drops tincture,   (1/4 part)

   or 1 tablet/cup) (1 part)   Ginger (1/4 part)

Gotu Kola (fresh tincture,

   1/2 part)

Note: The active ingredients of milk thistle, collectively called, *silymarin*, are not particularly water-soluble, so it is best to add a tincture or powdered extract of milk thistle to the finished tea.

Directions: Drink 1/8 to 1/2 cup of this decoction 3 to 5 times daily. Individual tinctures of the above herbs can be mixed in the proportions given to make an anti-addiction formula, if desired. Commercial herbal anti-addictive formulas are also available in natural food stores.

10. Protection Against Environmental Toxins

Diagnostic symptoms: Unexplained dizziness, ringing in the ears, nausea, fatigue, and "spaciness" can have a number of causes, but if they are experienced regularly, you should at least consider that sensitivity to chemical pollutants may be a factor. Toxic metals like lead and mercury are ubiquitous nowadays, having found their way into dental fillings and many other products, too. For a complete treatise on these issues, see Debra Dadd's excellent book, *Non-Toxic, Natural, and Earthwise.*

Dietary recommendations: As we've already discussed, most liver damage from environmental chemicals is thought to be due to excess free radicals. For this reason, it is good to add antioxidants and antioxidant containing foods to the diet. I recommend vitamin E, beta carotene, vitamin C, zinc, and selenium supplements (the latter two blended in a general nutritional supplement, not as an isolated single nutrient) during times of suspected toxic chemical stress. For regular maintenance, I suggest a program of spirulina (very high in beta-carotene), fresh greens, liver flushes, exercise and sweating, and other moderate cleansing measures, such as intestinal cleansing.

Another useful adjunct is fruit pectin powder, which has been used extensively in Russia for removing environmental toxins and radiation from the body. Take 1 to 3 tablespoons of the powder in water or fresh-squeezed fruit juice first thing in the morning and follow with two glasses of water or herb tea.

Bentonite clay is also useful. Put one teaspoonful in a glass of water, stir, and leave the mixture in the sun for a few hours to ionize the clay's micro-particles. When these particles are charged, they attract and bind toxins, thus helping to pass them from the body. One enema a day and saunas are also desirable during any cleansing.

Herbal recommendations: The herbal formula on the next page can be used in addition to the above measures. It invigorates bile flow, protects and detoxifies the liver, and stimulates phagocytosis to dispose of poisonous chemicals. I call this formula "Environmental Safe-Tea."

Environmental Safe-Tea

Milk thistle tincture
    (1 dropperful)

Echinacea root (1 part)

Fenugreek (1/2 part)

Yellow dock root (1/8 part)

Fennel (1 part)

Bladderwrack (1 part)

Burdock (1/4 part)

Ginger (1/4 part)

Oregon grape root
    (1/8 part)

Directions: Sweeten to taste with stevia herb or a little licorice. Decoct together in the usual way and drink 1/2 cup 2 to 3 times a day.

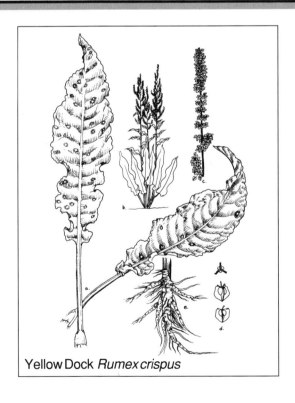

Yellow Dock *Rumex crispus*

General Guidelines
for Building Liver Vitality

- Lower your fat intake. Eat less refined, cooked oils and fats. Obtain essential oils from whole nuts and seeds.

- Rest the digestive system whenever possible. Don't eat too late at night or too early in the morning. Don't eat when not hungry, and especially never overeat.

- Be aware of proper food combining. Sweet fruit and cooked protein are the worst combination, causing fermentation.

- Liver flushes and drinking lemon-water keep the liver moisturized and free-flowing.

- Keep the eliminative channels open and free. Exercise to eliminate toxins via the lungs and skin. Have two bowel movements a day.

- Massage the liver area at least once a day to help remove congestion.

- Worry or anger can get stuck in the liver. Release these emotions in a constructive way.

- Antioxidants such as vitamins E and C, beta-carotene, zinc, and selenium protect against toxins. Herbal antioxidants are superior to synthetic vitamins (in my opinion), though both can be used together.

- Herbal formulas to cleanse, protect, and stimulate the liver are highly recommended. Try a tea of roasted dandelion, chicory, and ginger; Puri-Tea; Polari-Tea; or one of the other teas discussed in this section. Milk thistle is a must for rebuilding the liver when it has been compromised or weakened in any way.

The Herbal

The second half of this book consists of a reference list of important liver and digestive herbs, with in-depth information for each. Herbs are listed in alphabetical order (short descriptions of other useful digestive herbs not discussed in this main list can be found at the end of Chapter 5). Although this present list is by no means comprehensive, it does summarize and synthesize useful information gathered from a variety of sources, including from Traditional Chinese Medicine (TCM), Traditional European Medicine (TEM), and the traditional medicine of India (Ayurveda), as well as from modern chemical and pharmacological data and my own experience as an herbalist.

ANGELICA
(*Angelica archangelica* L., other *Angelica* species)

PARTS USED — The dried roots, the dried sliced roots (as in Dong Quai), and the dried seeds

BOTANY, DESCRIPTION, AND HISTORY OF USE — Angelica is a genus in the parsley family (Umbeliferae or Apiaceae). Its relatives include cumin, fennel, lovage, and celery. A number of angelica species were important Native American remedies for colds and digestive problems. The classic European angelica is *Angelica archangelica*, which is the most commonly used species in Western herbalism and is included in commercial products such as bitters. This

210

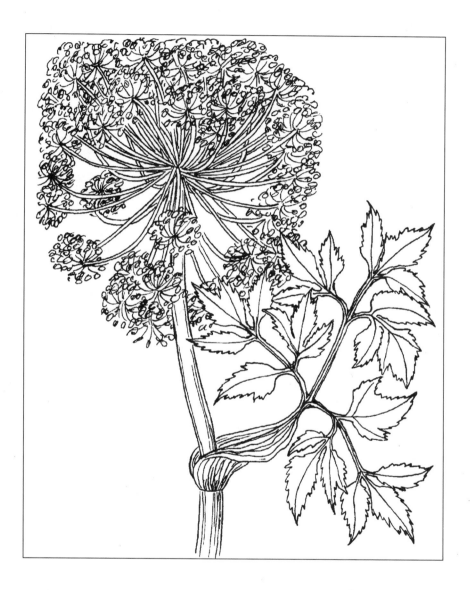

Angelica — Angelica archangelica L.

species has a long history of use. During the Middle Ages, it was used as a protector against plagues and poisons and as a remedy to help digestion after overeating. In China, many angelica species have been used as medicine for thousands of years; the roots of *Angelica sinensis* are processed to create the Chinese drug Dong Quai.

RELATED MEDICINAL SPECIES — There are a number of types of wild angelica growing in the United States which can be used for medicine—for instance *Angelica hendersonii*, common on the Pacific Coast.

ENERGY, TASTE, CONSTITUTIONAL PROPERTIES — In both TCM and TEM angelica is considered spicy, warming, drying, dispersing, thinning (as for mucus), and bitter. Dong quai moistens yin (builds blood); enters the lung and stomach meridians; and is opening and dispersing for the liver. Angelica is a *specific* herb (or *tonic*, depending on how it is processed.)

CONTRAINDICATIONS — The raw root is best avoided because it is rich in coumarins which can over-sensitize one to light and act as an anti-coagulant. Also, it is not indicated for constitutionally weak people with heat (infections) or diarrhea.

CHEMICAL CONSTITUENTS AND PHYSIOLOGICAL ACTIVITIES — *Angelica archangelica* is rich in coumarins, which are anti-coagulant compounds, and a complex volatile oil which has anti-bacterial and anti-fungal properties. These plants are used for many purposes, in a variety of cultures both East and West, but generally have stomachic, decongestant, and warming qualities.

SPECIFIC USES — Angelica is one of the best bitter tonic ingredients, and it is added to many formulas because it is bitter, spicy, and aromatic. It is also used to flavor liqueurs, baked goods, and other foods.   The warming attributes of angelica help moderate and balance the bitter taste of gentian and other bitter herbs. Add fennel, artichoke, and a little ginger and licorice to angelica to make an excellent digestive aid.

PREPARATIONS, FORMULAS, AND DOSES — Angelica root and seed are used in a number of European bitter tonic formulas (these are also available in the United States). In these formulas, angelica is generally mixed with gentian, sweet or bitter orange peel, rhubarb, centaury, artichoke, cardamon, licorice, and other digestive herbs. Four grams of angelica a day in decoction with other herbs (as above) is sufficient, or with a liquid extract, take about 35 drops 2x/day, before protein or fatty meals.

NOTES — Make sure to dry wild angelica before use, as it contains psoralens and coumarins (drying seems to mitigate the potentially irritating qualities of these compounds). I have harvested several wild American species and used them in my formulas with good results. Although these wild species need more clinical testing, they appear to have an excellent potential. *Angelica archangelica* makes a beautiful garden plant and is not difficult to grow when fresh seed is obtained. The seeds, especially, can be dried and macerated for two weeks in brandy or wine (and then removed), along with the other digestive herbs mentioned above, to make homemade bitters and digestive tonics.

ARTICHOKE
(*Cynara scolymus* L.)

PARTS USED — The leaves, fresh or fresh-dried

BOTANY, DESCRIPTION, AND HISTORY OF USE — Artichoke leaves are from the familiar, edible artichoke plant, which is a member of the daisy family and a relative of the important liver herb, milk thistle.

RELATED MEDICINAL SPECIES — I consider the leaves, stems, and roots of other wild and weedy thistles, such as Italian thistle (*Carduus pycnocephalus*), bull thistle (*Cirsium vulgare*), Canadian thistle (*Cirsium arvense*), and milk thistle (*Silybum marianum*), to be liver tonics and nutritives.

ENERGY, TASTE, CONSTITUTIONAL PROPERTIES — The leaves are cooling, opening, bitter, and slightly aromatic. The herb enters the liver and gallbladder meridians. Artichoke is a *specific* herb.

CONTRAINDICATIONS — Artichoke is an excellent liver tonic and digestive herb, with few contraindications, though it may promote too much bile production when taken in excess.

CHEMICAL CONSTITUENTS AND PHYSIOLOGICAL ACTIVITIES — The bitter constituent of artichoke, cynaropicrin, reaches its highest levels in the plant just before flowering and again at seed maturity. Research has identified another constituent, cynarin, which shows strong bile-stimulating and liver-protecting properties.

SPECIFIC USES — Because of its pleasant bitter and aromatic

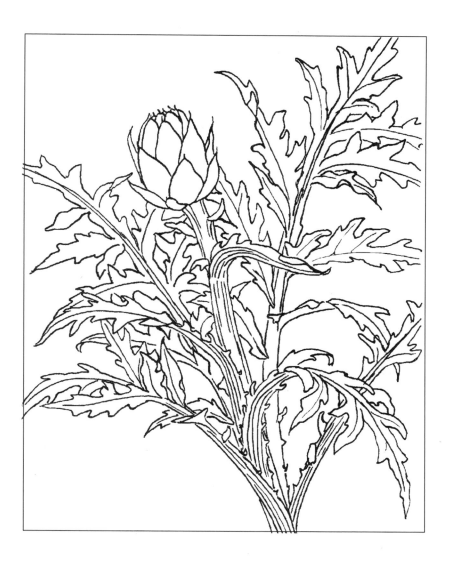

Artichoke — Cynara scolymus L.

quality, artichoke is one of the most widely used herbs in European bitter formulas. It is often mixed with gentian, bitter orange, cardamon, and other herbs to make commercial bitter formulas. According to Weiss (1988), artichoke is indicated for gallstone disease because of its cholesterol-lowering properties and may be useful for weight-reduction because it decreases the fat content of blood and increases digestive efficiency and elimination.

PREPARATIONS, FORMULAS, AND DOSES — Artichoke is commonly used in bitter tonics as an alcohol- or glycerin-based liquid formula which is taken in teaspoon doses just before or just after main meals (especially protein meals, as bitters stimulate the flow of hydrochloric acid, thus aiding digestion). If there are artichokes growing in your garden, use part of a fresh leaf, or a tablespoon of the dried leaf, to make a tea by simmering the herb in a cup of water for 10 minutes with one or two slices of ginger and a pinch of fennel seeds. Drink one cup of this tea morning and evening or around mealtimes.

NOTES — I have never smelled anything closer to buttered popcorn than the aroma of fresh or fresh—dried artichoke leaves. Despite these leaves' bitter flavor, artichoke preparations are pleasant, and one quickly develops a taste for them. I have found that preparations containing artichoke, milk thistle, skullcap, turmeric, and ginger are excellent for mild to moderate digestive upsets, inability to digest fatty foods, and to help relieve the unhappy effects of overeating. Bitter formulas are a must for many health imbalances, helping to relieve such symptoms as low energy and constipation. Bitters are also indicated for immune weakness, since artichoke and other bitter herbs (such as gentian) have been shown to stimulate immune function through sensors in the intestines.

BERBERIS, BARBERRY, OREGON GRAPE
(*Berberis aquafolium* Pursh., *Berberis* sp.)

PARTS USED — Roots, root bark, sometimes the ripe berries

BOTANY, DESCRIPTION, AND HISTORY OF USE —
Berberis, often called *Oregon Grape,* is a small perennial shrub of the barberry family (Berberidaceae). It has spiny leaves, lemon-yellow flowers, blue, edible berries and is widespread. Berberis is a common forest plant in the Pacific Northwest, and various other species grow throughout the world. In India, the root extract of *B. asiatica,* called Rasaut, is a popular home remedy as a digestive tonic, carminative, and blood purifier. The fruits are edible and are given to children as a laxative. In TCM, *B. thunbergii* is a Japanese folk remedy considered to strengthen the stomach, while *B. sargentainae* (Chinese barberry) is used to help clear jaundice, dysentery, eye irritation, and for external trauma. Both are considered cooling and are used for removing infections and soothing irritations in the digestive tract.

In TEM, the inner bark of *B. vulgaris* was well-known as a household remedy for jaundice and liver inflammations (hepatitis). In the United States, the Eclectic doctors often prescribed Oregon grape root (*B. aquifolium*) for easing chronic diarrhea, as well as for painful digestion accompanied by loss of appetite, due to the plant's duodenal activating properties. As in Europe with barberry, Oregon grape was known to help ease jaundice.

Also, Oregon grape was a popular remedy among Native American peoples who lived in California and Oregon. They made a decoction of the roots and drank it to alleviate general weakness and

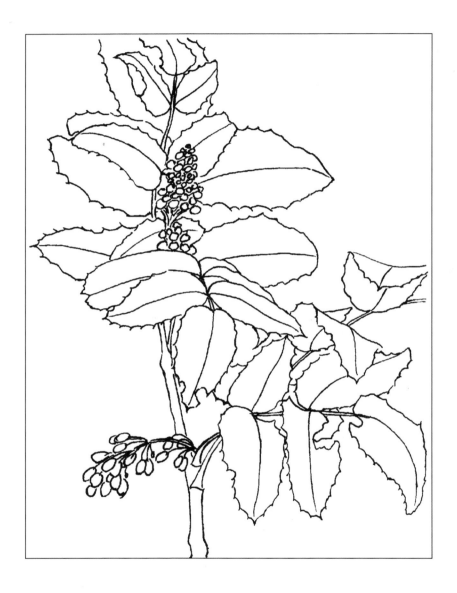

Oregon grape — Berberis aquifolium Pursh.

to help stimulate appetite.

RELATED MEDICINAL SPECIES — A number of berberis species are used in herbal medicine. *Berberis aquifolium* and *B. nervosa* are called Oregon grape; these species were important digestive and wound-healing herbs for the Native Americans. *Berberis vulgaris* is the European barberry, used as a dye plant; *B. canadensis* is the American barberry; *B. aristata* (or *B. asiatica*) is the Indian barberry; and *B. sargentainae* and *B. thunbergii* DC. are commonly used in China.

ENERGY, TASTE, CONSTITUTIONAL PROPERTIES — Berberis is bitter, slightly astringent, and cooling. It is a *specific* herb.

CONTRAINDICATIONS — When taken in large amounts or for protracted periods, berberis can contract and excessively cool the digestive tract. Berberine, a constituent of berberis, can affect the nervous system—but this should not be a problem when taking the whole herb in normal amounts. Use with caution or avoid during pregnancy.

CHEMICAL CONSTITUENTS AND PHYSIOLOGICAL ACTIVITIES — Oregon grape and other *Berberis* sp. contain the alkaloid berberine, which has a cooling, anti-inflammatory, and heat-clearing activity. Berberine is also bitter and stimulates the production of hydrochloric acid in the stomach, as well as the production of digestive and liver secretions in general. Other alkaloids in *Berberis* sp. include oxyacanthine and berbamine.

SPECIFIC USES — Berberis is used for liver fire (overheated liver); liver toxicity from drugs or alcohol; low stomach acid (poor protein assimilation); infections; or irritation in the intestines (irritable bowel syndrome or diarrhea due to irritation). Berberis can be of help with intestinal parasites such as giardia (combine it with black walnut, artemisia, garlic, or ginger for this purpose), or disordered intestinal bacteria (in which case take it with an acidophilus supplement 2-3 x/ daily). Berberis is also one of the best skin herbs for acne, psoriasis (combine it with milk thistle for this purpose), cysts, or sores—plus it is worth a try as an adjunct therapy for dandruff, along with cold water therapy and alternating shampoos.

PREPARATIONS, FORMULAS, AND DOSES — Berberis can be found in a variety of American, European, and Chinese formulas. The root powder, cut and sifted herb, and even pieces of the whole rhizome can be purchased in bulk. Berberis can be mixed with herbs such as ginger or prickly ash bark to help counteract its cool nature. Of the tincture, 20 to 40 drops (1 dropperful) morning and evening is a maintenance dose, while a dropperful morning, afternoon, and evening is a mild therapeutic dose. Of the capsules (powdered herb), take 2 capsules 3x daily. Of the powdered extract, take 100 to 200 mg 2x daily.

Or take a half-cup of the decoction morning and evening for up to 10 days. Berberis can be taken before or after fatty or protein-rich meals to help aid digestion.

NOTES — Oregon grape and other *Berberis* species can be used for a few weeks or up to two or three months because of their tonic properties. They are milder and have fewer side effects than golden seal (which contains hydrastine and affects the nervous system). Those who have white nails, frequent clear urination, and thin, watery mucus should always take berberis with ginger, fennel, or other warming herbs.

BLESSED THISTLE
(*Cnicus benedictus* L.)

PARTS USED — The herb, sometimes the seed

BOTANY, DESCRIPTION, AND HISTORY OF USE — *Cnicus benedictus,* the sole member of the genus, is from the thistle tribe in the daisy family (Asteraceae). A native of Spain and other parts of southern Europe, it is a beautiful, sprawling hairy thistle with bright yellow flowers. Blessed thistle is a well-known garden plant in many parts of the world.

Blessed thistle was known to the Greeks but was not much used by them as medicine, according to the herbals that survive. Pliny calls it *cnecos,* and says that the Egyptians held it in high esteem because of the useful oil they extracted from its seeds. Blessed thistle was known to and recommended by the Physicians of Myddvai (physicians to the Welsh royalty), starting around the middle of the 13th century. They prescribed the decoction for digestive pains. Blessed thistle was official in European medicine for a short time but fell out of favor with physicians in the early 1800s. However, it has remained a popular remedy until the present in European and American herbalism.

RELATED MEDICINAL SPECIES — None

ENERGY, TASTE, CONSTITUTIONAL PROPERTIES — Blessed thistle is considered sweet, cool, and slightly astringent in TCM. In TEM it is considered to be bitter, cleansing, opening, and hot and dry in the second degree. I consider it bitter and aromatic. It enters the liver meridian. Blessed thistle is a *specific* herb.

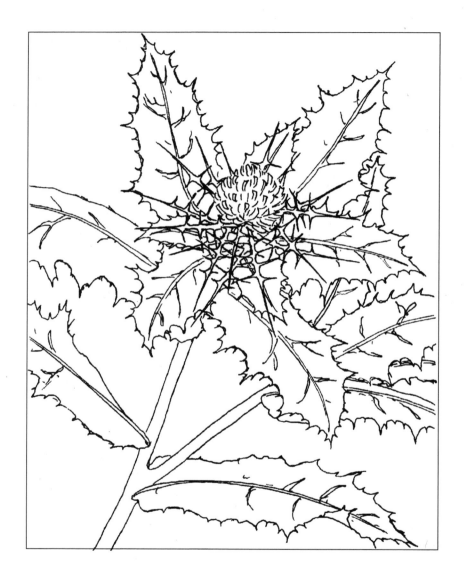

Blessed thistle — Cnicus benedictus L.

CHEMICAL CONSTITUENTS AND PHYSIOLOGICAL ACTIVITIES — Blessed thistle contains the sesquiterpene lactone cnicin, which is bitter and mildly antibiotic. It also contains lignans, phytosterols, volatile oil, tannins, mucilage, and mineral salts (especially potassium and magnesium, 10-18%). Blessed thistle is mildly astringent and stimulates bile flow and hydrochloric acid production.

SPECIFIC USES — Blessed thistle is recommended for anorexia and painful digestion. A cold infusion of the root can be helpful in debilitated conditions of the stomach, helping to restore appetite.

CONTRAINDICATIONS — Excessive quantities (over 3 or 4 cups of strong tea) may cause mild nausea in some people.

PREPARATIONS, FORMULAS, AND DOSES — Blessed thistle is available in bulk (leaf and stems), but avoid bulk powder. This herb is best in extract form, either as a liquid tincture or in combination with other herbs as a powdered extract. It combines well with aromatic herbs from the parsley family, such as fennel seed, caraway seed, or anise.

Dose: 5-10 drops in a little water or tea every 4 hours, up to a maximum of 25 drops 3 or 4 x/day. Make an infusion (1:20), and drink 1/3 to 1/2 cup cool or warm, 3-4 x/day.

NOTES — Blessed thistle is highly dependable in its action as a penetrating bitter and a liver and digestive tonic, but it should not be overused. Try starting with 5-10 drops per dose and working up to 20 or even 30 drops after a week. Take it in cycles of 10 days on, 3 off, and 10 on.

BUPLEURUM
(*Bupleurum falcatum* L., *B. chinense* DC., *B. scorzoneraefolium* Willd.)

PARTS USED — The root, either dried or stir-baked in honey, wine, or vinegar

BOTANY, DESCRIPTION, AND HISTORY OF USE — Bupleurum is one of several species of *Bupleurum*, a member of the Umbelliferae, or parsley family. These are slender plants with single alternate, parallel-veined lanceolate leaves and small umbels of yellow flowers. They commonly grow in grasslands in northern and central China and in other parts of Eurasia. The first test plantings in the U.S. were made in 1990 in Oregon.

Bupleurum is a traditional Chinese herb, first mentioned in the *Divine Husbandman's Classic of the Materia Medica* (25 to 225 A.D.). The Chinese name for this herb is Chái Hú, which means "kindling of the barbarians." The dry upper parts of the plant are said to have been used to start fires.

RELATED MEDICINAL SPECIES — One of 3 or 4 species (3 are listed above) traditionally have been used interchangeably in China.

CONTRAINDICATIONS — In some people, bupleurum in large amounts can cause nausea, in which case it is good to reduce the amount by half or more until it is tolerated. Try adding 1/2 part ginger and 1/4 part licorice to moderate this effect. Caution is also indicated in yin-deficient people with persistent coughs.

ENERGY, TASTE, CONSTITUTIONAL PROPERTIES — Bupleurum is bitter, slightly acrid, and mildly cooling. It enters the pericardium, liver, triple warmer, and gallbladder meridians, removing liver congestion, dispersing stagnation, and increasing the yang chi. The tea or concentrates are useful for relaxing constrained liver chi (helping with symptoms such as dizziness, vertigo, emotional excesses, and menstrual problems), and resolving disharmonies between the liver and spleen (accompanied by symptoms such as bloating, nausea, and indigestion). Bupleurum invigorates the spleen by enhancing the upward flow of vital energy and nutrients. It is a *specific* herb.

CHEMICAL CONSTITUENTS AND PHYSIOLOGICAL ACTIVITIES — The active constituents are considered to be saponin glycosides (saikosides, 2.8%), and also flavonoids such as quercetin, isoquercetin, isorhamnetin, rutin and narcissin, and volatile oil. In the laboratory, bupleurum has shown sedative, analgesic, anti-hepatoxic, antipyretic, antiviral (flu virus), and antitussive properties. The extract increases the total bile output, which helps remove toxins and digest fats.

SPECIFIC USES — This herb is excellent for restoring normal liver function, especially in patients with hepatitis, for which it is often prescribed either alone or in combination with other herbs. It is used in formulas that can help relieve painful digestion and early cirrhosis and remove heat from the liver (hepatitis, etc.).

PREPARATIONS, FORMULAS, AND DOSES — A decoction is made by adding about 10 grams of the herb by itself (I also add a little ginger and licorice), or about 20 grams total of a formula, to 12 ounces of water. Simmer the herbs for 45 minutes, strain off the liquid, add 6 ounces of fresh water, decoct for another 20 minutes, strain again, and then add the first liquid and store the tea in the refrigerator. Drink 1 cup of the tea in the morning and 1 in the evening. To check for individual tolerance, it is always best to start with 1/2 cup morning and evening for a few days, then build up to a full dose.

Several traditional formulas are very popular for various liver and gallbladder disorders, including the following (all amounts are in grams):

1. *Major bupleurum combination*: for gallstones, fatigue with sore liver, and tendency towards constipation, decoct bupleurum (6) with scutellaria (3), paeonia (3), ginger (4), unripe orange peel—chih-shih or Zhi Shi (2), jujube (3), rhubarb (1), and pinellia (3).

2. *Bupleurum and cinnamon combination*: for gallstones, gall-bladder inflammation, and loss of appetite due to intestinal discomfort, decoct bupleurum (5) with pinellia (4), licorice (1.5), cinnamon (2.5), scute (2), ginseng (2), paeonia (2.5), jujube (2), and ginger (1).

3. *Xiao yao wan (bupleurum sedative formula)*: see formula and indications on p.128.

NOTES — Bupleurum is one of the best-known Chinese herbs for harmonizing liver function and protecting it against stress.

BURDOCK
(*Arctium lappa* L.)

PARTS USED — The fresh or dried roots, and the seed

BOTANY, DESCRIPTION, AND HISTORY OF USE —
Burdock is from the Asteraceae, or daisy family. Its most noticeable
characteristic is its spiny flowering head, which sticks tenaciously to
socks and animal fur, spreading the seeds. Burdock is a biennial
herbaceous plant, producing a rosette of large wavy leaves the first
year and a tall, branched, flowering stalk the second. As a cultivated
plant, it is often treated as an annual, because the root and leaves are
best picked for food and medicine during the first year. I have seen
a single burdock plant that was eight feet high and very robust.

Burdock root is known as gobo in Japan, the seed as goboshi
(Japan) and Niú Bàng Zí (China). In TEM, it is known as lappa, the
great burre docke, or bardana.

RELATED MEDICINAL SPECIES — *Arctium minus*, a common weed, is also grown for medicine.

ENERGY, TASTE, CONSTITUTIONAL PROPERTIES —
Burdock is bitter and cooling. It enters the liver meridian and benefits
spleen deficiency. The seeds are most commonly used in Chinese
medicine, especially for skin problems. The roots are used in TCM and
Western herbalism as an alterative and digestive aid. In Japan, the roots
are used in cooking and medicine and are considered to strengthen and
tonify the spleen. Burdock is a *tonic* and *protective* herb.

CONTRAINDICATIONS — None known.

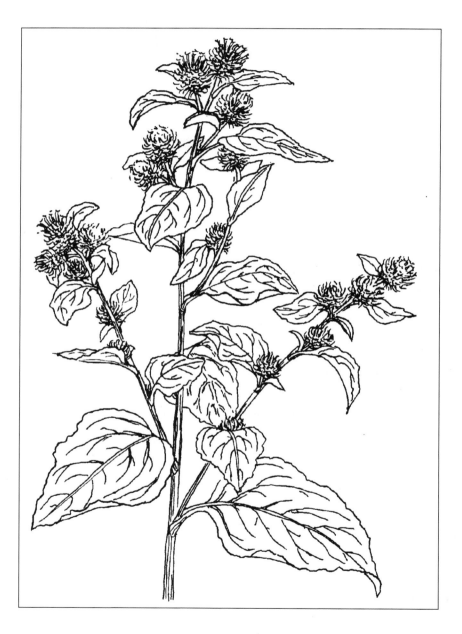

Burdock — Arctium lappa L.

CHEMICAL CONSTITUENTS AND PHYSIOLOGICAL ACTIVITIES — The plant contains, among other constituents, the carbohydrate inulin (ca. 50%), several polyacetylenes, tannin, polyphenolic acids (caffeic, chlorogenic, etc.), gobosterin, the sesquilignans, lappaol C, D, and E, the dilignans, and lappaol F and H. In 100 grams (2.5 ounces) of the fresh root can be found 61 mg of calcium, 77 mg of phosphorus, 1.4 mg of iron, 0.03 mg of thiamine, and 0.05 mg of riboflavin (Benoit, 1976). Modern research has isolated chemical constituents with anti-bacterial and anti-fungal, and most importantly, tumor-protective and desmutagenic properties. Desmutagens are defined as substances that inactivate mutagens (cancer-causing agents) by reacting with them and "taking them out of action." Burdock is also bile-stimulating, alterative and detoxifying.

SPECIFIC USES — This herb is recommended as a tea for cleansing programs. For acne and other skin problems (psoriasis), drink several cups of a strong decoction (1:5) of burdock and dandelion root (1:3). For liver stagnation and difficulty with fat digestion, the tea or powdered extract can be taken around mealtimes.

PREPARATIONS, FORMULAS, AND DOSES — Burdock is often recommended as a tea or powder. It is mixed with other roots, such as sassafras and dandelion, to make "root beer," a healing, delicious beverage for the liver and digestion (when it isn't made with refined sugar syrup). Combined with red clover, burdock is part of classic anti-cancer preparations—a use supported by modern studies.

NOTES — Burdock roots can be purchased in many natural food stores and even supermarkets. Slice them thinly and use them in stir-fries and soups. Burdock is also an important ingredient in many bowel-cleansing and lymphatic cleansing formulas.

CASCARA SAGRADA
Rhamnus purshiana DC.

PARTS USED — The aged (one year) bark of the branches and trunk

BOTANY, DESCRIPTION, AND HISTORY OF USE — Cascara sagrada is the sacred bark (*Rhamnus purshiana*) of many Native American peoples. The bark has been gathered for medicinal use for over 100 years and has been official in the United States pharmacopeia from 1890 to the present. The small trees grow abundantly from northern California to Alaska. The related *R. californica*, or coffee berry, is common in the coastal ranges throughout middle and southern California.

RELATED MEDICINAL SPECIES — *Rhamnus frangula* is the alder buckthorn of European herbalism..

ENERGY, TASTE, CONSTITUTIONAL PROPERTIES — Cascara sagrada is very bitter and slightly sweet; is cooling; and it stimulates digestive chi when taken in small to moderate amounts (less than 2 grams/day of the dried bark as a tea or in capsules). Cascara has both *tonic* and *specific* properties.

CONTRAINDICATIONS — It is not recommended for more than a few days of use for a person with hypertonic bowels (frequent, watery stools that have a short transit time), especially when there is immune weakness present.

CHEMICAL CONSTITUENTS AND PHYSIOLOGICAL ACTIVITIES — The herb contains about 10% anthraquinone glycosides, especially the cascarosides, but also quite a few others. All

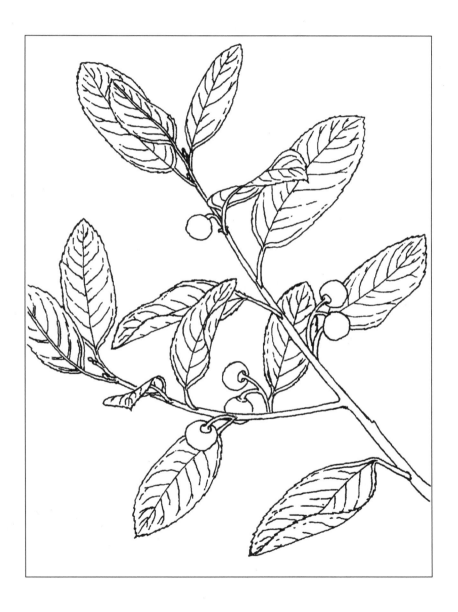

Cascara sagrada — Rhamnus purshiana DC.

of these stimulate increased peristalsis in the large intestine.

SPECIFIC USES — Cascara and its relatives are among the very best of the bowel tonics/laxatives, helping to re-educate bowels that are too lax or atonic. Its slightly sweet nature adds a nourishing, tonic quality to water-based preparations. While cascara is not known to be particularly habituating, any laxative used over a period of time (more than a few weeks) may diminish the natural tendency of the bowel to move. Cascara is too cold and bitter for people with profound immune weakness.

PREPARATIONS, FORMULAS, AND DOSES — Cascara is best used in combination with aromatic herbs, such as ginger, fennel, or cardamon, that can help counteract its cold, bitter nature (i.e., its tendency to cause contraction). Sweet herbs help enhance its tonic qualities and again help smooth out the bitter taste. I recommend adding 1/4 part licorice root to cascara formulas. If a definite laxative effect is needed where the bowel is very stagnant and sluggish, a stronger laxative containing 1/3 senna leaf or about 1/2 part rhubarb can be given for a time. Cascara was used as an elixir (a sweet, tonic, liquid herbal preparation) in times past and was tremendously popular. Essential oils of wintergreen, fennel, and other herbs were often added. The "official" preparation is the *Aromatic Cascara Fluid Extract*, which contains cascara, licorice extract, anise oil, coriander oil, wintergreen oil, alcohol, and water. The dose is about 5 ml.

NOTES — I have known people who have taken cascara formulas for months on end, in the belief that it helps tonify the bowel wall and improve elimination. It has a good reputation in this regard; however, I recommend that it not be used indiscriminately for over a week or so. Nonetheless, it is one of the best mild laxative—tonics available, and it increases the liver's ability to produce bile.

CHIONANTHUS OR FRINGE TREE
(*Chionanthus virginicus* L.)

PARTS USED — The root bark

BOTANY, DESCRIPTION, AND HISTORY OF USE —
Chionanthus, a member of the olive family (Oleaceae), is native to the
eastern United States. The name chionanthus is derived from the
Greek *chion* (snow) and *anthus* (flower) because of the beautiful white
appearance of the tree in bloom. Although it was used primarily by
most Native Americans for external purposes, the Cherokee, Dela-
ware, and Iroquois used the closely related American ash bark (*Fraxinus
americana*) as an important gastro-intestinal aid, laxative, and liver
aid. Chionanthus was prescribed for "portal congestion and the
treatment of catarrhal jaundice" (*U.S. Dispensatory* 25). The experience of the Eclectic doctor, John King, showed that it is an excellent
tonic for people recovering from long, debilitating illness. Because the
liver and digestion are so vital to health, they must be restored as
quickly as possible during convalescence. Thus, it is interesting to note
Felter and Lloyd's statement, "Chionanthus improves the appetite,
aids digestion, promotes assimilation, and is a tonic to the whole
system" (Felter-Lloyd, 1898).

In 1843, the Eclectic doctor Goss cured himself of jaundice using
this herb, which helped establish it as *the* standard remedy for jaundice,
as well as for other liver ailments. Scudder (1891) highly recommended the plant in 10-15 drop doses for gallstone attacks.

A few other digestive indications for which the Eclectics used
chionanthus include hypertrophy of the liver, chronic hepatic inflammation, or portal congestion; irritability of the stomach from "high

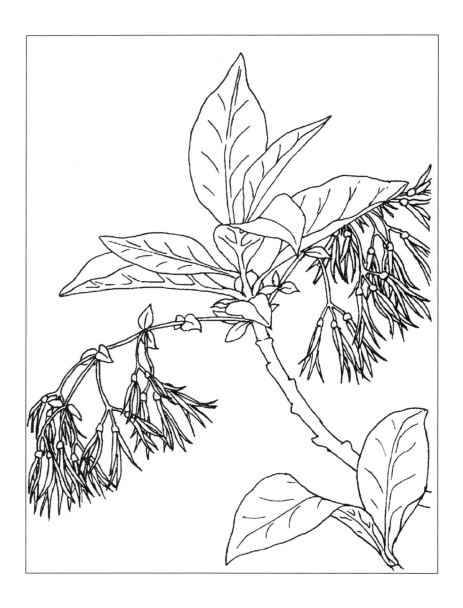

Fringe tree — Chionanthus virginicus L.

living" and the use of alcoholic stimulants; and inflammatory conditions of the duodenum. They also noted that it is worth trying in 2-5 drop doses for relieving colic in infants, and it may be useful for pancreatic disease.

RELATED MEDICINAL SPECIES — There are two species in the eastern United States and two in China, though there is little or no information on their uses. *Chionanthus retusus* has been studied for its chemical composition (Iwagawa, 1985).

ENERGY, TASTE, CONSTITUTIONAL PROPERTIES — Chionanthus is bitter and slightly aromatic; cool; and it removes congestion, especially from the liver and gallbladder. It is indicated for clearing heat and dissipating poisons from the liver. Chionanthus is both *tonic* and *specific*.

CONTRAINDICATIONS — Use this herb with caution in cases of deficient chi, or deficient spleen and stomach chi (i.e., weak digestion, in which case add spleen Qi tonic herbs such as astragalus).

CHEMICAL CONSTITUENTS AND PHYSIOLOGICAL ACTIVITIES — A bitter glycoside, chionanthin, and saponins have been found in Chionanthus. A Japanese species, *Chionanthus retusu*, contains the glycoside phillyrin ligustroside. Ligustroside is also a constituent of *Ligustrum lucidum*, a related species that is a major tonic herb for kidney yin deficiency and weakness of the sexual energy. Because chionanthus was used as a strengthening tonic by the Eclectics, the possibility that the herb has superior strengthening properties should not be overlooked. More clinical and laboratory work remains to be done.

SPECIFIC USES — According to *Hager's Handbook*, chionanthus is recommended as a homeopathic remedy for liver-related headaches and hepatitis. The herb extract is used for cirrhosis of the liver and jaundice. In general, the herb is used as a liver tonic for people who are not excessively deficient, where there is heat and congestion, especially venous congestion.

PREPARATIONS, FORMULAS, AND DOSES — Some Eclectic authors thought that the infusion or decoction was practically inert, much preferring the alcoholic extract or tincture.

NOTES — Chionanthus is probably one of the most useful and certainly underrated Native American liver herbs.

CHICORY
(*Cichorium intybus* L.)

PARTS USED — The steamed greens picked before flowering; the fresh and dried roots; the roasted roots; the seeds

BOTANY, DESCRIPTION, AND HISTORY OF USE — Chicory is a member of the Asteraceae, or daisy, family and is a close relative of dandelion. It was known and widely used for medicine and food by the ancient Greeks. Pliny mentions that "the juice of the boiled-down vegetable loosens the bowels, and benefits liver, kidneys and stomach....it benefits jaundice also if taken in honey wine, provided there is no fever."

It is native to Russia and most of middle and southern Europe and Eurasia. It was introduced into India at an early date. When I was in Greece, it was hard to find chicory greens because someone had always cut them off neatly at the ground before me. They are extremely popular as a delicious green vegetable dish called *horta*, which is prepared with olive oil and garlic. Also, roasted and chopped or ground root is extremely popular all over Europe as either a coffee substitute or as an admixture to coffee, because it has some of the same flavor components as coffee (chlorogenic acid and similar molecules).

RELATED MEDICINAL SPECIES — *Cichorium endivia* is the garden endive. It can be used like chicory greens but is more refined and less bitter.

ENERGY, TASTE, CONSTITUTIONAL PROPERTIES — The roots are mildly bitter and cold, especially when harvested in the late summer or in the fall. Spring roots are sweeter and more tonic

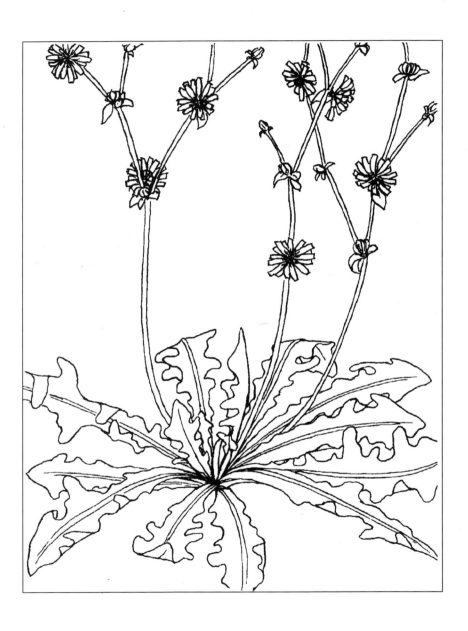

Chicory - Cichorium intybus L.

when picked before the above-ground parts develop. Chicory is tonic to the digestion and enters the liver and stomach meridians. The roots can help remove toxins and dampness from the blood, being especially good for "water toxins" that accumulate, especially during the winter, from eating too much raw vegetables and fruit. The concept of water toxins in TCM is difficult to interpret in Western terms, but may refer to either a condition in the body where there is too much water in the tissues or chemicals that are created in this overly-wet environment. Chicory roots are *specific*.

CHEMICAL CONSTITUENTS AND PHYSIOLOGICAL ACTIVITIES — Chicory contains the starch favorable to diabetics, inulin (up to 58%). The content is higher in the fall before the first frost, when inulin is broken down to fructose and other more simple sugars. The herb's bitter taste is due, at least in part, to sesquiterpene lactones, such as lactucin and lactupicrin. Chicory also contains the coumarins chicoriin, esculetin, esculin, umbelliferone, and scopoletin and sterols like taraxasterol. Research has shown the alcoholic extract to have anti-inflammatory effects *in vitro* (Benoit, 1976).

CONTRAINDICATIONS — Chicory is considered safe by most herbalists, but a 19th century French doctor said (Cazin, 1886) that chicory is indicated for bilious people who suffer from habitual constipation, but contraindicated for people whose vital energy reserves are depleted or who have a "lymphatic or bloodless persons." This may translate to "yin deficiency" in TCM. The Renaissance herbalists cautioned that taking chicory too freely or abundantly "causes venous passive congestion in the digestive organs within the abdomen and a fullness of blood in the head." I have not observed this and have known people, including myself, who have drunk a quart a day of the tea for a week with no ill effects. Lewis (1791) says that chicory can be taken freely and safely for inflammatory conditions and that it keeps "the belly open."

SPECIFIC USES — The root, when added to dandelion and/or burdock with a little ginger, makes a good cleansing tea that can be taken *ad lib* during a program of liver flushes, fasting, and sweating. Though mild, chicory can be added to liver herb formulas for more severe liver problems such as hepatitis. It is safe for children, acting as a mild laxative. Also, I often recommend chicory as a cleansing tea for skin eruptions, such as acne. For this purpose, mix it with dandelion, Oregon grape, and a little fennel, and drink 1 cup morning, afternoon, and evening.

PREPARATIONS, FORMULAS, AND DOSES — The decoction of the fresh, dried, or roasted root is preferred to the alcoholic extract. Chicory combines well with ginger, burdock, dandelion, and sassafras. Decoct 1 ounce of the root in 1 pint of water, and drink the resulting tea freely.

NOTES — Roasted chicory root is one of the best coffee substitutes for those trying to kick the coffee habit. Also, its slightly sedative and liver- and bile-promoting activity tends to ease the jittery withdrawal feelings that often accompany the elimination of coffee addiction.

CITRUS
Citrus aurantium L., *Citrus limon* (L.) N.L. Burm., *Citrus* sp.

PARTS USED — The peel of the unripe fruit, especially of the sweet orange, dried whole or in slices

BOTANY, DESCRIPTION, AND HISTORY OF USE — All species of citrus come from the citrus family, Rutaceae. Many are small trees with dark green, aromatic leaves and orange, green, or yellow fruits. Sweet oranges may have originated from China, where they are extremely abundant today and are widely used by herbalists for digestive and upper respiratory complaints.

RELATED MEDICINAL SPECIES — Citrus peels, other than from unripe oranges, (such as lemon and grapefruit peels, even when ripe) may be useful as additions to bitter tonics because of their aromatic, bitter, and tonic nature.

ENERGY, TASTE, CONSTITUTIONAL PROPERTIES — Unripe citrus peel can be considered a tonic herb with some specific actions. Like many aromatic herbs, it is warming to the surface and cooling to the interior. It is bitter and aromatic and sometimes mildly sweet. Constitutional indications are for weakened digestion, especially due to lack of digestive enzymes. Green citrus is *specific*.

CONTRAINDICATIONS — Use citrus with moderation for ulcers of the stomach, esophagus, or duodenum, or when any other state of hypertonicity of the digestive tract is present. Caution is recommended for individuals with deficient chi.

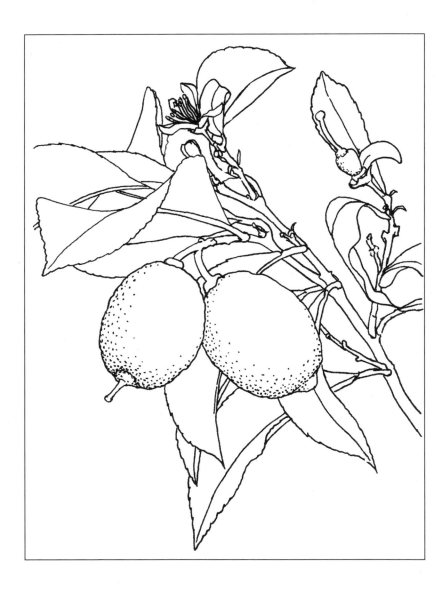

Citrus — Citrus limon (L.) N.L. Burm.

CHEMICAL CONSTITUENTS AND PHYSIOLOGICAL ACTIVITIES — The essential oil of citrus contains many terpenes, especially *d*-limonene, myrcene, camphene, pinene, and many others These have been shown to have a wide variety of physiological activities, including antibacterial, anti-inflammatory, and smooth muscle-relaxing properties.

SPECIFIC USES — Citrus peels are considered tonic to the digestive organs generally. They smooth the flow of the surface chi, especially when digestion is disordered due to lack of digestive enzymes. They also stimulate bile flow and gently remove liver stagnation. They are specifically recommended for use with gentian, artichoke, or other bitter herbs to help smooth the activity of these herbs, thus preventing the powerful increase of peristalsis and secretions that these herbs can induce when used by themselves.

PREPARATIONS, FORMULAS, AND DOSES — Citrus makes a wonderful tea: simmer a small handful of peels (2 ounces) in 10 ounces of water. You can add herbs such as ginger, cardamon, and fennel to make the tea more aromatic, gas-relieving, and warming; barberry, Oregon grape, or golden seal to make it more bitter and cooling (this helps clear heat, bringing immune force to the mucous membranes during infections); and gentian for more bile and liver stimulation.

NOTES — Although most people think of the sweet pulp when considering citrus fruits, the peels have more to offer in the way of healing properties. They contain flavonoids, such as neohesperidin, hesperidin, naringin, and others, which help strengthen connective tissue and especially blood vessels; and they also offer good anti-inflammatory and free-radical scavenging properties. One of the most overlooked benefits of citrus peels is their high content of pectin (about 30%, depending on season and type), which is an excellent detoxifier. Pectin is highly ionic and can draw and hold environmental toxins, radioactive compounds, and heavy metals and carry these out of the body. It is also an ingredient in commercial formulas, such as Kaopectate, which are widely used to mitigate diarrhea.

CYPERUS
(*Cyperus rotundus* L.)

PARTS USED — The dried tuberous rhizomes

BOTANY, DESCRIPTION, AND HISTORY OF USE — Cyperus is a member of the sedge family, Cyperaceae. The plant is commonly called "purple nut-grass" or "chufa" in English. It is a perennial with scaly stolons that terminate in edible tubers. It grows 6 to 20 inches high, has numerous narrow leaves, and umbels of thin, branched spikelets. It is a common weed in lower California (from the San Francisco Bay area to the border), as well as in the southeastern United States. Various species are common weeds in other parts of the world.

Cyperus has been considered an important medicinal plant from ancient times. In China it was used as a stimulant and stomachic and for normalizing depressed liver function. In India it was used to relieve constipation and gas. It was official in the first *Pharmacopeia Londinensis* (1618) and was said to have a warming nature and to provoke urination and the breaking of kidney stones.

RELATED MEDICINAL SPECIES — Many other species of *Cyperus* have been used in TEM, TCM, and Ayurveda, especially *C. esculentus, C. longus,* and *C. odoratus.*

ENERGY, TASTE, CONSTITUTIONAL PROPERTIES — In TEM, cyperus was considered mildly warm, bitter, and sub-astringent. In TCM, it is thought to be pungent, mildly bitter, and neutral and is said to enter the liver and triple-warmer meridians. In Ayurveda, it is pungent and bitter and relieves kapha conditions.

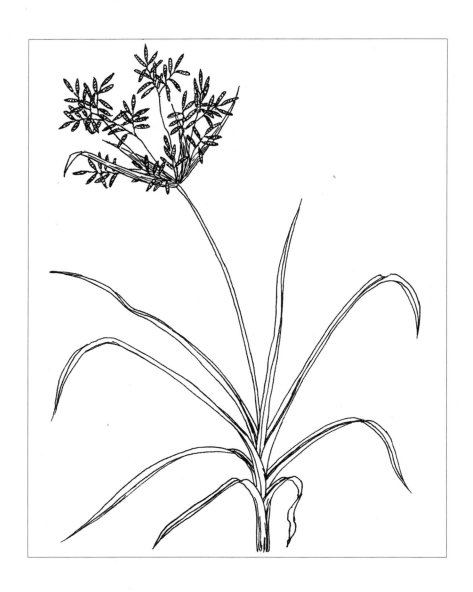

Cyperus — Cyperus rotundus L.

In TCM, cyperus is often used to "regulate the flow of vital energy and relieve stagnancy of a depressed liver, regulate menstruation and relieve pain" (Zhicen, 1987). The herb is also recommended when there is a disharmony between the liver and spleen, with bloating, epigastric pain, and tenderness of the upper abdominal or liver area. Cyperus is *specific*.

CONTRAINDICATIONS — Use cyperus with caution for individuals with deficient chi or deficient yin. The herb may also be estrogenic, in which case it is contraindicated for breast cancer and PMS (Bensky and Gamble, 1986).

CHEMICAL CONSTITUENTS AND PHYSIOLOGICAL ACTIVITIES — Cyperus contains about 0.5-1% essential oil (a complex mixture of mono- and sesquiterpenes, such as cyperene, cyperol, etc.); 0.21-0.24 alkaloid; 0.62-0.74% cardiac glycosides; 1.25% flavonoids; 1.62% polyphenols; and sugars, starch, and pectin (4.21%).

According to *Hager's Handbook*, it is used as a diaphoretic, diuretic, gravel-remover, carminative, astringent, as a remedy for liver ailments, as an emmenagogue, for dysentery, and as a stimulant and tonic.

SPECIFIC USES — Cyperus is recommended for pain in the liver and bowels, hardness and pains in the epigastrum, and emotional stagnation. For hepatitis, combine it with turmeric and milk thistle. Cyperus is also used for amenorrhea and other menstrual difficulties, when these are not due to excess estrogen, as well as for postpartum headache.

PREPARATIONS, FORMULAS, AND DOSES — The usual TEM dose is 5 to 7 grams in decoction. In TCM, 4.5-12 grams is decocted as a daily dose. According to Bensky and Gamble, soaking the cyperus tubers in vinegar and drying them increases the herb's ability to enter the liver channel and treat pain.

NOTES — This herb is much underrated. It is a gentle, warming, and stimulating tonic that has tremendous value for treating many kinds of liver and digestive disorders.

DAN SHEN
(*Salvia miltiorrhiza* Bunge)

PARTS USED — The roots are cultivated in China, where they are dug up in the spring or autumn and cleaned and dried for use.

BOTANY, DESCRIPTION, AND HISTORY OF USE — The plant is a member of the genus Salvia from the Labiatae, or mint family. It has been highly revered in China since ancient times and is considered to be one of the "five astral remedies" (Wu-shen) which were thought to correspond to the five colors and five principal organs. Specifically, dan shen is red and is associated with the heart and liver. It was recommended in TCM for moving blood, removing congestion, and as a sedative.

RELATED MEDICINAL SPECIES — There are over 600 different species of *Salvia* world-wide, according to some estimates. Many of these are used in cooking and medicine. Often it is the aromatic upper leaves and shoots that are sought for their warming, expectorant, and cough- and sore throat- relieving properties.

ENERGY, TASTE, CONSTITUTIONAL PROPERTIES — Dan shen is bitter and slightly cold in TCM. It enters the heart and liver meridians; moves blood, thus relieving stagnancy (congealed blood); protects the liver and helps relieve constrained liver chi; is sedative; and is useful for menstrual disorders. Dan shen is specific.

CONTRAINDICATIONS — Because of dan shen's powerful blood-moving properties, it is advised that this herb be used cautiously when the blood is not congealed. "Congealed blood" means that the blood is obstructed or circulation is slowed—generally due to hypertonicity of the sympathetic nervous system, or degenerative obstructions such as fatty deposits or sclerotic lesions in the vessels or perhaps leakiness of the vessels.

CHEMICAL CONSTITUENTS AND PHYSIOLOGICAL ACTIVITIES — Dan shen contains a series of phenanthranequinones, such as tanshinone I, IIa, IIb, and cryptotanshinone, as well as salviol and vitamin E. Research shows that dan shen extracts may dilate blood vessels, allowing increased blood, nutrient, and oxygen flow to tissues and organs, especially the liver and heart. Thus, dan shen can relieve ischemia and enrich nutrition and regenerative processes. Clinical tests show that over 70% of patients with chronic hepatitis respond to dan shen therapy: liver function tests improve, and subjective symptoms of nausea, weakness, and abdominal distention are relieved. Dan shen is *specific*.

SPECIFIC USES — Dan shen may be combined with skullcap, mugwort or capillaris, ginger, burdock, and/or other liver and gallbladder herbs for hepatitis, cirrhosis, or enlarged and sore liver (i.e., one with blood stagnation).

PREPARATIONS, FORMULAS, AND DOSES — Often prepared as a tea (1:20), dan shen is also available as a liquid and powdered extract as a single herb or in combination formulas. The usual dose is 3-15 grams per day.

Traditional Chinese formulas containing dan shen are not often mentioned in the Western literature on digestive and liver complaints. It is modern clinical and laboratory work that has highlighted the herb's ability to protect and move blood in liver conditions.

NOTES — Also called red-root sage, dan shen is vigorous and easy to grow commercially.

DANDELION
(*Taraxacum officinale* G.H. Weber ex Wigg.)

PARTS USED — The fresh, dried or roasted root, and the fresh or dried leaves

BOTANY, DESCRIPTION, AND HISTORY OF USE — Dandelion is a close relative of chicory and is a member of the daisy or Asteraceae (formerly Compositae) family. The plant grows in most parts of the world and is said to be indigenous to Tibet. Dandelion is a common lawn and waste-lot weed and is available in many places at many times of the year. It has a basal rosette of large-toothed leaves that are 2 to 8 inches long and bright yellow heads of ray flowers borne singly on hollow stalks.

Various species of dandelion were known to the ancients in both the West and the East. See my complete monograph on dandelion for a complete account of the history of use, cultivation of, and research on this herb (Eclectic Medical Publications, Portland, OR; 1989).

The first certain references to dandelion's use as medicine come from Arabian physicians of the 10th and 11th centuries (Levey, 1966). By the 15th century, dandelion was well established in European apothecary shops (Grieve, 1931; Faber, 1958), where it became popular as a liver herb for everyday use. Culpeper (ca. 1660) wrote that dandelion is "under the dominion of Jupiter" and that it is valuable for "removing obstructions of the liver, gallbladder, and spleen and diseases arising from them, such as jaundice."

In India, dandelion root has been used and cultivated for unknown centuries as a valuable liver and digestive remedy and food.

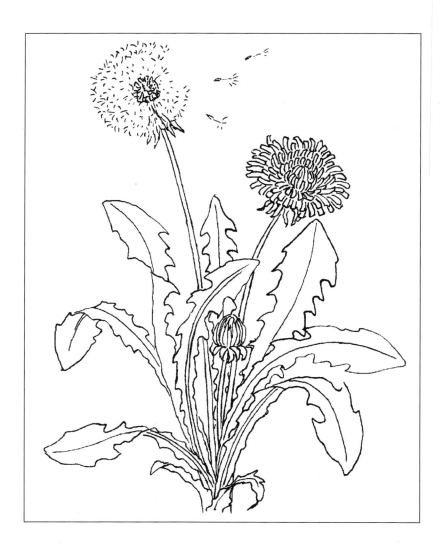

Dandelion — Taraxacum officinale G.H. Weber in Wigg.

In TCM, it was mentioned in the *Pen T'sao* as a detoxifying herb, especially useful for cooling liver fire and clearing abscesses or sores.

RELATED MEDICINAL SPECIES — Many other species of dandelion are used world-wide for medicine and food. The number of species of *Taraxacum* is not agreed upon by botanists, but most herbalists feel that they are all equally medicinal.

ENERGY, TASTE, CONSTITUTIONAL PROPERTIES — Dandelion has a cold nature and a bitter taste and should be used in decoction for clearing fevers, detoxifying the system, and for cooling heat conditions in the liver, digestive organs, and skin (boils, abscesses, swellings, etc.). In the winter and spring, the root is sweet, tonic, and more neutral in nature. Harvested at this time, it is useful for helping to stabilize blood sugar and mood swings—though it is still a good tonic for the liver. Dandelion roots harvested in the summer and fall tend to be *specific*, while winter and spring roots are more *tonic* and *protective*.

CONTRAINDICATIONS — This herb is very safe and can be taken in large amounts for moderate lengths of time—for example, in 10 day cycles, up to 3 or 4 months. If the root is very bitter, it is best to moderate its cooling and contracting effects with a bit of ginger and licorice.

CHEMICAL CONSTITUENTS AND PHYSIOLOGICAL ACTIVITIES — Dandelion root contains simple and complex sugars, such as inulin, pectin, and mucilage; the coumarin derivatives coumesterol, scopoletin, and esculin; many flavonoids; tannins; fatty acids; a small amount of essential oil; sesquiterpenes such as lactucin and lactupikrin (bitter components); and a number of steroid compounds, such as the pentacyclic compounds taraxasterol and beta-amyrin.

Recent Chinese medical studies on liver and gallbladder disease seem to corroborate the traditional view that herbal formulas containing *Taraxacum* are curative due to their bile-promoting and anti-microbial effects. Dandelion has also been proven to be effective in treating appendicitis—a disease that in traditional Chinese medicine is diagnosed as an imbalance of the liver and gallbladder organ systems—*without* surgery (C.P. Li, 1974). Finally, dandelion coffee has a sweet flavor and is highly aromatic because the roasting process breaks down inulin into fructose and also releases many aromatic principles. The drink gently stimulates the digestive and eliminative organs, and, unlike caffeinated coffee, is neither addictive nor harmful to the body.

SPECIFIC USES — Take dandelion as a tea as much as you wish for cooling irritations and infections of the liver. The herb is also excellent in formulas for hepatitis, cirrhosis, and liver toxicity. It has a tendency to lower blood cholesterol levels with continued use. Both the traditional use and modern research point toward an anti-carcino-genic activity, especially for breast cancer. One cancer-protective compound in dandelion was shown to be a glucose polymer similar to lentinan (from shiitake), called TOf-CFr. Also, dandelion has demonstrated estrogen-lowering capabilities. Medical science is currently accepting the connection between excessive levels of estrogen and breast cancer—and in holistic thought, it is the liver that must clear excess estrogen and thus reduce the risk of cancer.

PREPARATIONS, FORMULAS, AND DOSES — Dandelion root is best prepared as a tea (1:10) by simmering it for 20 minutes, then steeping it for 10 minutes. Drink 1 cup 2-5 times daily if you tolerate it well. You may drink dandelion alone or mix it with sweet and slightly aromatic herbs, such as cyperus, licorice, ginger, or fritillaria. You may also mix it with cool and bitter herbs, such as forsythia fruits or chrysanthemum flowers (*C. indicum*), to enhance dandelion's detoxifying and heat-clearing ability.

NOTES — The lowly dandelion is one of the best day-to-day remedies for cooling and strengthening the liver. When the liver is overworked from processing heavy emotions, environmental or endogenous toxins, or heat of pathogenic origin (virus, bacteria, etc.), dandelion is a safe and effective remedy. Also, its nutritional value is excellent, since both the roots and leaves are rich in nutrients and minerals.

FRUIT, UNRIPE (PLUMS, APPLES)
Prunus domestica L.

PARTS USED — Green, unripe plums or apples; whole fruit, either fresh or dried

BOTANY, DESCRIPTION, AND HISTORY OF USE — The green, unripe fruits recommended here are produced by members of the rose family (Rosaceae). They are all small trees that are commonly cultivated in many parts of the world. These fruits are thought to have originated in Asia Minor but were known to the Greeks and Romans.

RELATED MEDICINAL SPECIES — Any species of apple, plum.

ENERGY, TASTE, CONSTITUTIONAL PROPERTIES — Unripe plums and apples are bitter, sour, astringent, and neutral to warm. They are indicated for deficiency conditions of the stomach and liver or gallbladder, because they stimulate the production of digestive enzymes. These fruits are also traditionally used in TCM to eliminate worms and check diarrhea because of their astringency. In Greece, unripe plums are given to promote good digestion. Unripe plums and apples are *specific*.

Unripe tangerine peels are considered bitter, acrid, and slightly warm in TCM; they have an affinity for the liver and gallbladder and help release and smooth the free flow of liver chi and reduce pain. They also help relieve food stagnation and gas.

CONTRAINDICATIONS — Use unripe plums and apples carefully in excess conditions, especially with hypersecretion of digestive enzymes and hydrochloric acid. Do not eat more than 1/2 to 2 small fruits, otherwise overstimulation of digestive secretions, cramping,

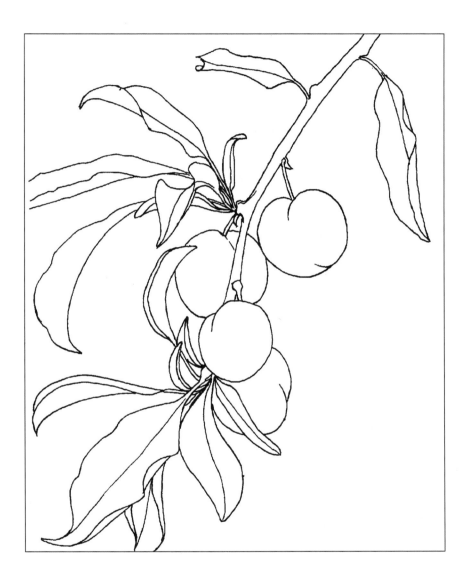

Unripe plum — Prunus domestica L.

and stomachaches may result. Caution is recommended for individuals with deficient chi.

CHEMICAL CONSTITUENTS AND PHYSIOLOGICAL ACTIVITIES — Unripe plums and apples are rich in fruit acids such as citric, malic, and succinic acids. They also contain phenolic compounds and hydrolyzable tannins, which help increase hydrochloric acid levels. In my experience, unripe fruit is preferable to giving hydrochloric acid tablets, which may weaken the body's ability to produce its own.

SPECIFIC USES — Use unripe fruits for digestive weakness due to deficient enzyme, bile, and acid production; trouble digesting protein and fat foods; inability to gain weight due to poor assimilation; food stagnation (slow transit time, abdominal swelling and pain) and gas.

PREPARATIONS, FORMULAS, AND DOSES — Unripe fruits are best eaten in their fresh state, 1 to 2 small fruits per dose, especially in season (spring) to help remove waste accumulation and digestive stagnation from the winter. To make a tea (1:10), simmer unripe plums or apples lightly for 10 minutes, then steep them for 10 minutes and drink 1/2 cup, as needed. Plums and apples can be mixed with coptis and skullcap for treating diarrhea due to pathogens (dysentery, giardia, bacteria)—though they are often used alone for this purpose.

NOTES — Children instinctively eat unripe fruit, though parents usually warn them against it, saying that the fruits will "give you a tummy-ache." However, if not taken in excess, unripe fruits from the rose family (especially plums and apples) can actually help children build good digestion. During a trip to Greece, I was intrigued to see push-cart vendors selling unripe plums. Dishes with these small, green fruits were often brought to the table after meals.

GENTIAN
(*Gentiana lutea L., G. macrophylla* Pall., *G. kurroo*, Royle, *G.* sp.)

PARTS USED — The whole dried root, either in slices or cut and sifted

BOTANY, DESCRIPTION, AND HISTORY OF USE — Gentian is one of several species from the genus *Gentiana* from the gentian family (Gentianaceae). Gentians are usually high mountain plants with vivid blue or yellow flowers and opposite leaves.

In TCM, gentian was mentioned as early as the *Pen King*—200 B.C. to 200 A.D.—and is thought to have been used in even more ancient times.

In TEM, Dioscorides recommended a cold-water infusion of gentian (the roots were crushed first) to help liver and stomach complaints. Galen thought it excellent for cleansing and removing obstructions. Gentian was an important ingredient in the famous anti-poison formula, *Theriaca*, perhaps because of its ability to re-move liver fire (toxic irritation or inflammation) and support the cleansing and detoxifying capabilities of the liver. Gerard (1633) said of it, "The decoction drunke is good against the stoppings of the liver, and crudities of the stomach, helps digestion, dissolves and scatters congealed blood, and is good against all cold diseases of the inward parts." Culpeper thought that gentian was one of the principal herbs ruled by Mars and that it "strengthened the stomach exceedingly...and [can] open obstructions of the liver and restores...appetite."

In Ayurveda, a type of gentian, probably *Gentiana chirayita* (Roxb.) or *G. kurroo* Royle, was considered a tonic and stomachic.

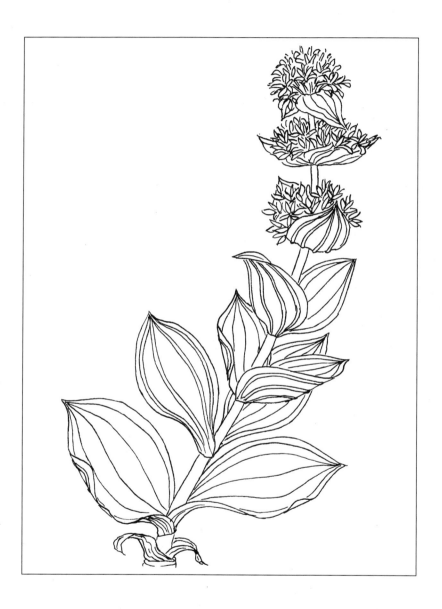

Yellow gentian — Gentiana lutea **L.**

RELATED MEDICINAL SPECIES — Many species of gentian are used throughout the world. In the United States, a number of species are harvested and made into various extracts for the commercial herb market. I have experimented with a number of California species and have found them to be uniformly bitter and sweet and excellent digestive aids.

ENERGY, TASTE, CONSTITUTIONAL PROPERTIES — In Ayurveda, gentian is considered to alleviate kapha conditions and poisoning. In TCM, it is deemed to be bitter and cold, entering the liver and gallbladder channels and is used to drain damp heat from the liver and gallbladder. In TEM, gentian is considered bitter and hot. According to Maiwald (1987), it is indicated for convalescence and exhaustion and "in general for constitutionally-created weaknesses." The seeming contradiction between TCM and TEM can be explained by the fact that gentian activates the flow of digestive juices, including hydrochloric acid and in that sense is heating; however, it can also alleviate inflammation and irritation in the liver and gallbladder and thus is cooling. Gentian is *specific* and mildly *tonic*.

CONTRAINDICATIONS — Gentian is cold and contracting when used too frequently or in doses excessive for one's constitution.

CHEMICAL CONSTITUENTS AND PHYSIOLOGICAL ACTIVITIES — The plants are rich in the bitter-tasting iridoid glycosides, amarogentin, gentiopicroside, and swertiamarin, and also xanthones, alkaloids (gentianine and gentialutine), phenolic acids (gentisic, syringic, and sinapic acids), sugars, and a small amount of volatile oil. Laboratory and clinical studies have shown that gentiopicroside and gentian extract can stimulate gastric secretion of enzymes, increase bile flow, and produce an anti-inflammatory effect.

SPECIFIC USES — Gentian is good for weak and/or painful digestion, loss of appetite, slow peristalsis, low vital energy, liver heat, detoxification, and acne. It is also used as an anti-addiction herb (for instance, for stopping smoking).

PREPARATIONS, FORMULAS, AND DOSES — The best-known way to take gentian is in combination with other herbs as a "bitter," just before or after a meal. It is also possible to make a tea with gentian by simmering 1 part root pieces in 20 parts of water for 20 minutes. To make a basic tea formula, mix 1/2 part gentian with 1 part organic orange, tangerine, grapefruit, or lemon peel, or any combination thereof—though I have found that orange or tangerine alone tastes the best with gentian when combined with 1/2 part fresh ginger root.

Compound gentian tincture was official in the *United States Pharmacopeia* until 1950 and in the National Formulary until 1960. The compound contained 10 parts of gentian, 4 parts bitter orange peel, and 1 part cardamon seed. To make this formula on your own, macerate the herbs (100 grams gentian, 40 grams bitter orange peel, 10 grams cardamon) in 900 ml of 100 proof vodka mixed with 100 ml of vegetable glycerin. Let the maceration proceed for 2 weeks, shaking the jar daily. Then, press or squeeze the liquid out, and filter if desired. The usual dose is 4 ml.

Another official preparation was the "glycerinated Gentian Elixir." I have modified the formula for this preparation so that it can be made at home. Follow the recipe below, using ready-made tinctures, or use the same proportions of cut and sifted herbs (in grams). If some of the tinctures are not available, take the same number of grams of the cut and sifted herb, grind it to a powder in a blender, and soak it in just enough 100 proof vodka to cover it. Keep the jar in a warm place out of direct sunlight, shaking every day for two weeks. Filter the pure liquid, discard the herb, and it is ready for use.

Digestive Power Formula

Gentian — 10 ml

Dandelion — 15 ml

Caraway seed — 15 ml

Cardamon seed — 25 ml

Cinnamon — 20 ml

Raspberry syrup — 60 ml

Sweet orange peel — 15 ml

Vegetable glycerin — 400 ml

Honey — 200 ml

100 proof vodka — 250 ml

NOTES — Gentian is probably the most popular of the bitter tonic herbs. One can find it in bitter tonic formulas such as "angostura bitters" in liquor stores and in many patent formulas sold in natural food stores. Although gentian has an extremely powerful and lingering bitter taste, it can be moderated with aromatic or spicy herbs, such as ginger, cardamon, or orange peel. Also, it has an intrinsic sweet taste that makes the harshness of its bitter taste less objectionable and more tonifying. The first time I tried straight gentian extract, I took quite a large dose of pure liquid extract without diluting it. To my surprise, immediately I felt powerful, regular waves of muscular activity in my digestive tract from head to rear. This lasted about 5 minutes, and afterwards, I enjoyed excellent digestion during my evening meal!

One important consideration when using gentian (and bitters in general) is the length of time you take it. The longer the use (up to several months or even years), the greater the benefits. See the section on bitters (in Chapter 5) for a more complete explanation of bitters.

GINGER
(*Zingiber officinalis Roscoe*)

PARTS USED — The fresh or dried rhizome, either whole, cut and sifted, or in powder

BOTANY, DESCRIPTION, AND HISTORY OF USE — Ginger is a member of the tropical family Zingiberaceae. The genus contains about 60 species, several members of which are used for medicine. The plant grows up to 3 feet or more in height, with narrow 6-12 inch leaves. The yellow flowers are in 2-3 inch spikes. Ginger is probably native to the Pacific Islands but is cultivated in many countries, including China and India. It has been used since antiquity in TCM, TEM, and Ayurveda. It was used by the Romans and has been popular down through the ages in many parts of the world for its flavor and warming properties. Dioscorides said that it was "good for the stomach."

RELATED MEDICINAL SPECIES — Many species are culti-vated and used for medicine and flavoring food, including *Z. cassumunar* Roxb., *Z. chrysanthum* Rosc., *Z. elatum* Roxb. in India, *Z. amaricans* Bl. in Java, *Z. purpureum* Roxb. in Laos, and *Z. zerumbet* (L.) Sm. and *Z. mioga* (Thunb.) in China.

ENERGY, TASTE, CONSTITUTIONAL PROPERTIES — In TCM, ginger is considered to be spicy and warm and is used in about half of all prescription formulas. It is widely used to warm and disperse cold, especially in the spleen, stomach, lungs, and kidney. The herb works well with people who are deficient and cold. Bensky and Gamble (1986) report that it is recommended for "pallor, poor

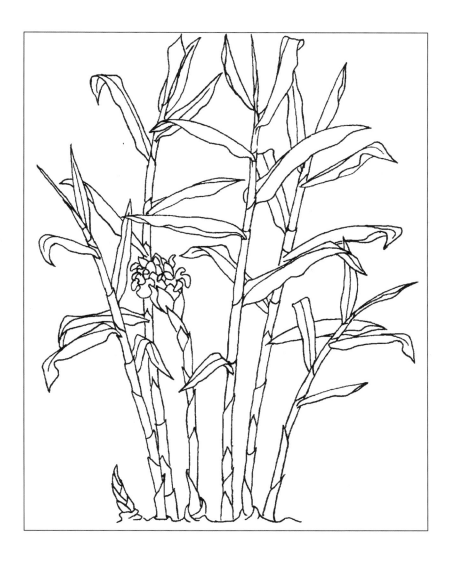

Ginger — Zingiber officinale

appetite, cold limbs, vomiting, diarrhea, cold painful abdomen and chest, a deep, slow pulse, and a pale tongue with a moist, white coating." They also say that it is known to "rescue devastated yang and expel interior cold with such signs as very weak pulse and cold limbs." A distinction is made between the fresh and dried rhizome. The fresh one is recommended for nausea, coughs, and gas, while the dried one is used for abdominal pain, lower back pain, and diarrhea.

In Ayurveda, ginger is used to alleviate kapha and vayu conditions and to cure constipation, diarrhea, obstruction to the movement of wind from the stomach, and the pain of colic.

In TEM, ginger is said to "heat and dry in the third degree" (Gerard, 1633). It was used in Europe throughout the ages to alleviate painful digestion, flatulence, colic, and diarrhea and as an ingredient in bitters formulas. Ginger is *specific* and mildly *tonic*.

CONTRAINDICATIONS — Because of its great warming powers, ginger should be used cautiously with people who are already hot-natured, especially where there is yin-deficiency. Although ginger is often recommended for alleviating the nausea of morning sickness, it should be used in moderation during pregnancy.

CHEMICAL CONSTITUENTS AND PHYSIOLOGICAL ACTIVITIES — Ginger rhizome contains a complex essential oil (1-3%), the pungent constituents gingerols and shogaols, and phenolic compounds. When ginger is fresh, the gingerols predominate, but during drying, the gingerols are formed, which are about twice as pungent. For this reason, dried ginger is more warming.

The herb is carminative, antispasmodic, and relieves nausea and coughs. It also activates the circulation in various organs and systems, and clears stagnation from bio-energetic channels.

SPECIFIC USES — Because of its superb anti-cramping qualities, ginger is one of the best remedies for muscle spasms in the stomach or intestines. These spasms can be quite painful and often result from overactivation of the sympathetic nervous system due to stress with no proper physical outlet. In these cases, make a tea from fresh or dry ginger, and drink it throughout the day as needed.

Ginger is also excellent as a tea, powder, or liquid extract for digestive stagnation (slow transit time), painful digestion, painful gas buildup, and in formulas for liver ailments such as hepatitis, cirrhosis, or gallbladder disease. It makes an excellent addition to the morning liver flush (see the section on liver flushes in Chapter 6).

PREPARATIONS, FORMULAS, AND DOSES — Ginger is best used by making a decoction from the fresh or dried rhizomes, which are readily available in most natural food markets (organic, of course) and herb shops. Simmer 1:10 for 20 to 30 minutes, and drink 1/2 to 1 cup several times daily, or as needed. One can also buy candied ginger, pickled ginger, ginger candy, ginger syrups for coughs and digestive problems, as well as a wide variety of other patent formulas.

For general use, as with nausea, intestinal spasms, gas, and as a general digestive aid, take 1 to 2 dropperfuls of the liquid extract (in a little warm water or tea), or 2 to 4 capsules of the dried herb, morning and evening as needed.

NOTES — I am very fond of ginger and use it in about 75% of my own commercially-marketed and custom formulas. I regularly use pickled ginger (available where macrobiotic foods are sold, often in markets in the international section) as a digestive aid and condiment during meals, and fresh-squeezed ginger juice when I take a morning liver flush.

GOLDEN SEAL
(*Hydrastis canadensis* L.)

PARTS USED — Usually the dried rhizome is used, but the leaves and stems are sometimes used as well.

BOTANY, DESCRIPTION, AND HISTORY OF USE — The genus *Hydrastis* is from Ranunculaceae, or the buttercup family, and contains 2 species, golden seal from eastern North America and another species from Japan. Golden seal is a shade-loving woodland perennial. It grows to 1 foot high and has rounded, 5-9 lobed leaves up to 8 inches across. The flowers are inconspicuous (1/3 inch) and greenish-white, and the fruit is berrylike and crimson-colored.

Golden seal is truly an herb of the Native American people. It was unknown in Europe until the middle or late 1800s, when its uses were taught to the European settlers as a sign of friendship. The herb was widely used by the indigenous people of the eastern United States for many ailments, especially as a wash to heal inflamed or infected eyes, and as a digestive and liver remedy. The Catawbas boiled the root for jaundice and chewed a piece of the green or dried root to relieve the stomach. The Cherokee used golden seal as a bitter digestive tonic. And the Iriquois used it as a carminative, gastro-intestinal aid, and a liver aid.

Golden seal was very popular in frontier and Eclectic medicine and was recommended by some of the great medical doctors and naturalists of the time, including Rafinesque, who used it as a stomach and liver remedy; Elisiah Smith, who used it as a laxative and for painful digestion; Horton Howard, who used it for loss of appetite; and

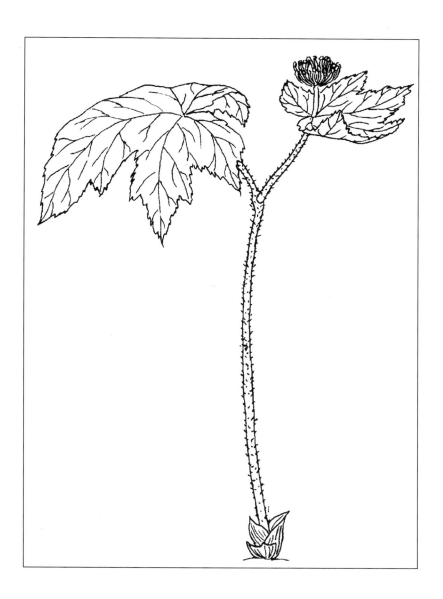

Golden Seal — Hydrastis canadensis L.

Samuel Thompson, who used it for indigestion and as a bile corrector.

RELATED MEDICINAL SPECIES — The Japanese species is *H. jezoensis,* Sieb.

ENERGY, TASTE, CONSTITUTIONAL PROPERTIES — Golden seal is bitter and cold. It enters the liver, stomach, and large intestine channels. It is detoxifying, drying, and cools the stomach. Small amounts of the herb stimulate digestive chi (especially when mixed with other warming herbs), but large amounts dampen it. Golden seal is *specific* and mildly *forcing.*

CONTRAINDICATIONS — Do not use this herb with people who have deficient yin, and use it cautiously in deficient spleen or kidney syndromes. Golden seal should be used only in moderate amounts and for cycles of 10 days on, then 10 days off, for no more than 2 complete cycles at a time. It tends to contract and cool the digestion excessively in people who are deficient or weak, especially when taken in amounts over 2 or 3 "00"-size capsules a day for one 10-day period. The herb should not be used during pregnancy, as it is a uterine stimulant (I have seen large amounts cause abortion).

CHEMICAL CONSTITUENTS AND PHYSIOLOGICAL ACTIVITIES — All parts of the plant, but especially the rhizome, contain several alkaloids, namely hydrastine, berberine, and canadine. In the Western view, these compounds are considered alterative to the mucous membranes and are bitter tonics. Golden seal is often recommended to lower inflammation, nourish surface tissues, and regulate mucous secretions from the gastrointestinal tract, urinary tract, and upper respiratory tract. In the laboratory, the alkaloid berberine demonstrates a cholagogic effect and can stimulate bile production and reduce its viscosity. It also lowers serum cholesterol.

SPECIFIC USES — Bensky and Gamble recommend golden seal for chronic cholecystitis. It is especially useful for chronic excess mucus in the bowels, with attendant loss of efficiency in absorbing nutrients and eliminating wastes. It is also often helpful when a person has a diet rich in mucus-forming foods, such as rich refined dairy product-containing foods with wheat and eggs. In this case, golden seal can help expel mucus and can alleviate irritation. Because of its bitter tonic qualities, golden seal is useful in small amounts for irritation in the bowel where the tone is poor and there is lack of appetite and painful digestion.

PREPARATIONS, FORMULAS, AND DOSES — Golden seal powder is often taken in "00"-size capsules or as a 1:5 liquid tincture at 20-30 drops per dose, 2-3x /day for up to 10 days. The herb is found in many formulas for colds, flu, upper respiratory tract infections, and digestive problems.

NOTES — Golden seal has gone through several periods of high popularity in the United States and is still one of the best-selling herbs of all time. Unfortunately, because of constant high demand, it has been wiped out in many areas where it formerly flourished. Organically-grown plants are now available in limited supply at a higher price.

MILK THISTLE OR MARY'S THISTLE
(*Silybum marianum* [L.] Gaertn.)

PARTS USED — The ripe seeds or an extract of the shell only

BOTANY, DESCRIPTION, AND HISTORY OF USE — The genus *Silybum* is a member of the thistle tribe of the daisy family (Compositae). There are two species, both native to southern Europe and Eurasia, one of which is *Silybum marianum*. Milk thistle is a stout thistle: I have seen it grow up to 12 feet tall in rich well-watered soil. The flowering heads are bright purple, large (up to 6 inches in diameter), and beset with very sharp spines. The leaves are milky-banded, hairless, and succulent when young, the only protection being a row of prickles on the margins. Milk thistle seeds and roots have been used since antiquity for digestive and liver complaints.

RELATED MEDICINAL SPECIES — There is one other species, which is used similarly to *S. marianum*, though rarely, *S. eburneum*.

ENERGY, TASTE, CONSTITUTIONAL PROPERTIES — Milk thistle seeds are nutritive, slightly bitter, and sweet and tonic to the liver, spleen, and kidneys. They are indicated for constitutional liver or spleen weakness and are taken long-term (up to 9 months). Dioscorides extols the remedy for protection against snake bites. In TEM, Galen (A.D. 155) wrote that the seed "is of a thin essence and hot facultie." Culpeper (1650) wrote of its effectiveness for removing obstructions of the liver and spleen. In popular German herbalism, milk thistle has a long history of curing jaundice and other liver disorders. This, no doubt, helped stimulate modern German research into the plant, which has established it as a widely prescribed

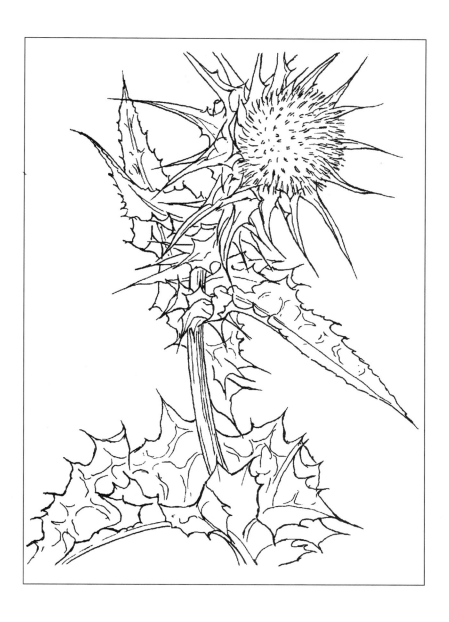

Milk Thistle — Silybum marianum [L.] Gaertn.

modern phytomedicine for liver disease. The genus does not seem to be known in TCM or Ayurveda. The whole seeds are *tonic*, while the purified, standardized extract is *specific, tonic,* and *protective*.

CONTRAINDICATIONS — None known.

CHEMICAL CONSTITUENTS AND PHYSIOLOGICAL ACTIVITIES — The extensive modern clinical and laboratory research on milk thistle seed would fill (and has filled) a whole book. The most important active constituents discovered thus far are the flavonoid-like compounds called *flavanolignans,* the group of which is collectively called *silymarin.* The three most abundant of these molecules are silbinin, silychristin, and silydanin. These compounds, have two major actions: 1.) They bind to the liver cell (hepatocyte) membranes and protect them from being injured by foreign chemicals, endogenous and environmental toxins (such as death-cap mushroom toxins), and free-radical damage; and 2.) They enter the liver cells and enhance their ability to produce enzymes vital to the liver's proper functioning, thus speeding recovery from injury to the liver and even stimulating regeneration of liver tissue. The seeds are also rich in betaine, a proven liver protector, as well as essential fatty acids that may help lower excessive and chronic inflammation in the body.

SPECIFIC USES — Use this herb for protection and enhanced liver regeneration after exposure to heavy metals, radiation, or toxic chemicals. Milk thistle is an important part of a therapeutic regime for hepatitis (both chronic and acute) or cirrhosis. It is also useful for psoriasis or other skin ailments, according to clinical experience.

PREPARATIONS, FORMULAS, AND DOSES — Silymarin is not particularly water-soluble, so it is best to take milk thistle in a liquid or powdered extract form, though some people enjoy eating the seeds or cooking with them as a mild liver and nutritive tonic. The herb is also finding its way into many patent formulas for the liver and digestion. The usual dose of the unstandardized liquid extract is one dropperful (40 drops) 2 or 3 times daily; of the powdered extract standardized to 10% silymarin, it is up to 100 mg 2 or 3 times daily; of the powdered extract standardized to 80% silymarin, it is 1 or 2 tablets daily.

NOTES — I first learned of milk thistle in early 1984, when I began harvesting seeds from wild plants growing in California and taking the liquid extract I made from them. I had sustained heavy damage to my liver as a result of having hepatitis twice, in 1963 and in 1967, and I was able to greatly restore my digestive power with the help of this herb. Since then, I have witnessed other surprising recoveries from severe liver ailments with the use of this herb.

MUGWORT AND WORMWOOD
(*Artemisia douglasiana* Bess., *A. vulgaris* L., *A. capillaris* *Thunb.*, *A. californica* Less., *A. absinthium* L.)

PARTS USED — The tops of the plant in flower or the leaves

BOTANY, DESCRIPTION, AND HISTORY OF USE — Artemisia is a large genus (about 200 species) from the daisy family (Compositae), mostly from the arid regions of the northern hemisphere. The name comes from *Artemis*, a Greek goddess of healing. Many artemisias are grown in gardens for medicine, for their beauty, and as food additives. Several kinds were and still are used as ritual plants as smudge and for external heating applications (moxa). The plants are herbs or small shrubs and are usually aromatic. The leaves are variable, often dissected, but usually covered with white hairs. The flowering heads are small and inconspicuous, having elongated, branched spikes.

Mugwort has long been used as a common folk-remedy in England for "hysteria" and menstrual disorders, and on the continent, especially in Germany and Italy, as a bile stimulant, bitter tonic, and antispasmodic.

RELATED MEDICINAL SPECIES — Many artemisias have been used for medicine over the millennia. In TEM, herbs like *A. dracunculus* L. (tarragon), *A. abrotanum* L. (southernwood), *A. annua* L. (sweet annie), and *A. absinthium* L. have been used for flavoring food and drink as well as for medicine since antiquity. In TCM, *A. apiacea* Hance is used as a liver and gallbladder herb for clearing summer heat, and *A. capillaris* is used for clearing damp heat

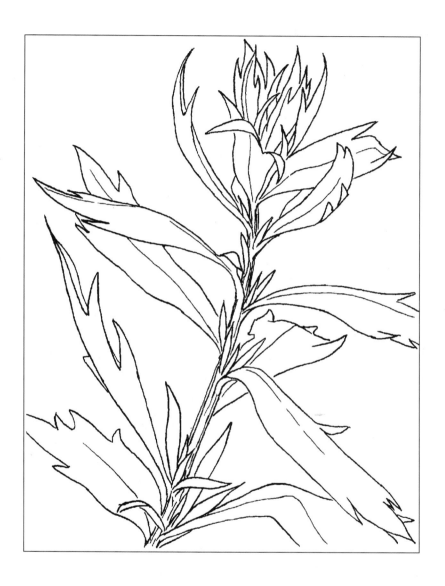

Mugwort — Artemesia douglasiana Bess

from the gallbladder and liver. In Ayurveda, *A. gmelinii* Weber ex
Stechm. (seu *A. sacrorum* Ledeb) is used for abdominal pains, and *A.
maritima* var. *thomsoniana* C.B. Clarke is recommended as a stomachic and laxative.

ENERGY, TASTE, CONSTITUTIONAL PROPERTIES — In
TCM, mugwort is considered bitter and cool, entering the liver,
spleen, gallbladder, and stomach meridians. It is the most important
herb for treating jaundice from damp heat or damp cold. In Ayurveda,
several species were used—many grow in northern India, in the
Himalayas—for their benefits to the digestion. I consider mugwort
bitter, aromatic, and neutral, and a *specific* herb.

CONTRAINDICATIONS — Mugwort is much milder than other
Artemisia species; consequently, I have observed no problems with its
use. Modern pharmacognosists say that mugwort, wormwood, and
other *Artemisia* sp. contain essential oil components (thujone) that
may be harmful when purified and given in large amounts, but there
are no reports of human toxicity with mugwort. As an example of how
much of *Artemisia tridentata* (a kind of sagebrush, which I consider
to be stronger than mugwort) must be eaten by range animals before
any symptoms are noticed, one reads in Kingsbury (a standard reference) that "sage sickness" develops in horses "previously unaccus-
tomed to sage, within a few days after being placed on a sagebrush
range. Symptoms include nervousness, and a tendency to fall when
moved...due to partial paralysis of the forelimbs. Nothing more
serious develops, and after a week or two, the horses are able to
consume large quantities of sand sage without developing further
symptoms." Remember that we are talking here about eating very
large quantities of the plant, as the sole or at least a major component
of the diet. Mugwort is not mentioned in one of the most comprehen-

sive works on the toxicity of plants, *Giftpflanzen* (Roth, et al., 1984), and Weiss (1988) says that mugwort is "much weaker" than wormwood.

The essential oil of wormwood is toxic, and its use can lead to serious nervous disorders. However, Weiss notes that the bitter principle of the herb is not toxic, and that the "usual wormwood preparations contain so little of the oil that there is no risk of toxic effect."

CHEMICAL CONSTITUENTS AND PHYSIOLOGICAL ACTIVITY — Mugwort, and all *Artemisia* sp., contain complex volatile oils and sesquiterpenes as well as flavonoids and phytosterols. In Western herbalism, the plant is considered emmenagogic, diaphoretic, choleretic, diuretic, stomachic, and useful as a medicine against worms. It is used in infusion for painful digestion and menstruation.

SPECIFIC USES — Mugwort is one of the best mild bile-promoting herbs. It is used as a tonic when there is difficulty digesting fatty or protein foods and as a general remedy for mild indigestion. Weiss (1988) recommends wormwood as "a proven stomach and gallbladder remedy...It relieves the lesser symptoms of atonic and achylic states in the stomach...and ameliorates the sensation of fullness and cumulation of gases...It is one of our best remedies for biliary dyskinesia or a gallbladder apt to cause trouble." He further states that wormwood is one of the most useful herbs for people recovering from illness, especially following influenza, because it helps to invigorate digestion and restore energy. Asthenics (people who have a constitutional condition characterized by spells of fatigue, digestive weakness, and pain in the stomach or gallbladder area, which are usually brought on by physical strain, emotional stress or excitement, or excessive eating) also benefit from wormwood. Finally, wormwood drops are a good standby remedy for gallbladder patients or dyspepsics (for this purpose, take 20 drops in 1/4 glass of water).

Wormwood is a very common European remedy but has not caught on much in the United States. If wormwood is not available, use mugwort, which has similar but weaker properties.

PREPARATIONS, FORMULAS, AND DOSES — Wormwood is often used in TCM formulas with bupleurum to drain excess fire from the liver and gallbladder. Bensky and Gamble (1986) mention that capillaris is less drying and "softer" than bupleurum for this purpose and that it is "especially useful when people with deficient yin constitutions or excess fire need the heat-clearing effects of bupleurum, but are unable to tolerate its dry nature."

NOTES — For years, I have eaten a leaf or two of mugwort during the spring, summer, and fall, while going on walks through the woods near my house. I find that it is refreshing and that it helps to stimulate my digestion, normalize bowel and liver function, and eliminate excess emotion that may be stuck in my liver or gallbladder. I have the Pacific Coast mugwort, *A. douglasiana* here, but I have tasted many others throughout the United States and Europe and have found them comparable. I highly recommend a leaf now and then, if the plants grow nearby; or pull up a bit of the rhizome and plant it in your garden at home.

RED ROOT
(*Ceanothus americanus* L., *Ceanothus* sp.)

PART USED — Root bark, root slices, fruits

BOTANY, DESCRIPTION, AND HISTORY OF USE — This shrub is from the buckthorn family (Rhamnaceae), the same family as cascara sagrada. Several species are used in herbal medicine. In the eastern United States, *C. americanus* is the classic "red root," so called because the root has a rich, red color. The Native Americans used this herb extensively as a remedy for diarrhea and other bowel complaints and considered it to be strongly astringent.

RELATED MEDICINAL SPECIES — In the western United States, several species were used in medical practice by the Eclectic doctors—e.g., *C. interrigimus*, *C. velutinus*, and *C. thrysiflorus* (California lilac)—as blood purifiers and cleansing herbs. Red root is a New World remedy; it was not known in Chinese or Ayurvedic medicine.

ENERGY, TASTE, CONSTITUTIONAL PROPERTIES — Red root is a good astringent bitter. It is cooling and increases circulation, but may be drying to mucous membranes (surface). Red root is a *specific* herb.

CONTRAINDICATIONS — This herb is not the remedy of choice for damp heat in the liver (hepatitis).

CHEMICAL CONSTITUENTS AND PHYSIOLOGICAL ACTIVITIES — Red root contains mainly alkaloids, such as ceanothine and others. Several species have been tested and shown to contain different alkaloids. It also has triterpenoid acids such as

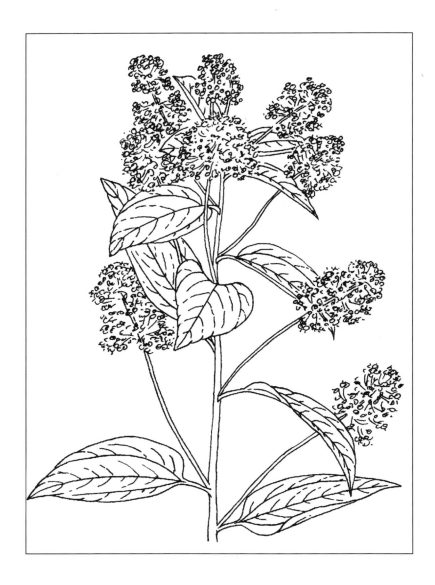

Redroot — *Ceanothus americanus L.*

betulinic acid, ceanothic acid, etc. Methyl salicylate is reported in some species, and I have distinctly smelled it in several California species, including *C. thyrsiflorus*.

According to Moore (1979), red root helps increase the efficiency of waste transport from the lymph to the liver. This may be why this herb is often recommended with liver and bowel cleansing programs, because it helps the liver do its job. Little scientific work has been done with this genus, but *Hager's Handbook* reports that *C. americanus* has a mild blood-pressure lowering activity.

SPECIFIC USES — Red root is an excellent cleansing herb. It is traditionally said to be a lymph cleanser and is one of the first cleansing herbs an herbalist uses, along with poke, ocotillo, and echinacea. Ellingwood called red root one of the best remedies for chronic congestion of the liver (stagnation), especially when portal circulation is impaired. He used it for "lymphatic patients" with sallow skin, puffy and expressionless faces, pain in the liver or spleen with hypertrophy of either or both organs, and constipation.

PREPARATIONS, FORMULAS, AND DOSES — The liquid extract of the root bark is excellent. Take 25-40 drops of it 2 or 3 times a day. A few days of red root can be helpful during cleansing fasts (with liver flushes), especially when the liver area is congested or mildly sore, or during any cleansing programs, such as sweats or colon cleansing. The root slices can be added to fennel to make an anti-congestive liver tea. Take 1/2 cup of this tea 2 times daily.

NOTES — Red root can be purchased in an herb store or natural food store. The western species can be harvested by pulling up one or two roots from a shrub and carefully cutting them (using stout cutters, for the roots are tough) and replacing the dirt. Make longitudinal slices and dry for use, or use the roots fresh.

SCHISANDRA
(*Schisandra chinensis* [Turcz.] Baill.)

PARTS USED — The dried, ripe fruits

BOTANY, DESCRIPTION, AND HISTORY OF USE —
Schisandra chinensis is a vine from the schisandra family, Schisandraceae, which is closely related to the magnolia family. It originates from the mountains of northern China and has been an important tonic remedy since ancient times. The vine grows upon trellises, like hops. It has thin, lime-green, serrate leaves; small creamy flowers; and small, round, bright red fruits. The remedy is considered a superior tonic in TCM and has been written about since around the time of Christ (in the *Pen King*).

RELATED MEDICINAL SPECIES — A total of 25 species occur, mainly in Asia, but one of these, *S. coccinea* Michx., grows in the eastern United States. Some of the other Asian species are used medicinally (Perry, 1980). The fruits of *S. grandiflora* are used in India but are not considered a major remedy there.

ENERGY, TASTE, CONSTITUTIONAL PROPERTIES — In TCM, schisandra is regarded as being sour and warm, though the Chinese name, *wu wei tsu* means "five flavors berry." In the *Su Kung* (7th century), it is said that "the skin and the pulp of the fruit are sweet and sour, the kernels are pungent and bitter, and the whole drug has a salty taste." It is indicated for "loss of essence," frequent urination from deficient kidneys, and deficiency of the spleen. It is also recommended as a folk medicine in Korea for promoting digestion. Schisandra is *tonic,* with some *specific* and *protective* properties.

CONTRAINDICATIONS — Caution is advised for excess heat syndromes; otherwise, it is generally considered safe.

CHEMICAL CONSTITUENTS AND PHYSIOLOGICAL ACTIVITIES — Several constituent groups in schisandra have demonstrated marked liver-protective ability in the laboratory, namely, lignins (schisantherin D, wuweizisu C, and gomisin A) and tannins. In one test with 102 patients with infectious hepatitis, a cure rate of 76% was noted when powdered schisandra fruit was administered (Bensky and Gamble, 1986).

Modern research has shown that schisandra berry extracts act as adaptogens, helping to restore proper harmony during stressful times, and that they also increase stamina and endurance.

SPECIFIC USES — Use schisandra with other adaptogenic herbs, such as eleuthero (*Eleutherococcus senticosus*) or ashwaganda (*Withania somnifera*), for people who are recovering from illness or who have depressed adrenal function due to stress. Because of the balanced flavor profile of this fruit, it is recommended for mild digestive or liver disorders, especially when caused by stress or overwork.

PREPARATIONS, FORMULAS, AND DOSES — This herb occurs in a great many Chinese patent formulas, as well as formulas available in the United States for dieting, energy, sports, and some digestive formulas. The usual dose is 6-9 grams in decoction.

NOTES — I love the expansive taste of dried schisandra fruits and often carry them in my pocket. Judging by people's reactions over the years in classes when I have passed these fruits out, they are very well liked.

TURMERIC
(*Curcuma longa* L.)

PARTS USED — The fresh or dried rhizome

BOTANY, DESCRIPTION, AND HISTORY OF USE —
Turmeric is a member of the ginger family (Zingiberaceae) and the genus *Curcuma*, which contains about 50 other species. The name comes from the Persian *kurkum*, meaning "saffron", because of the bright yellow color of the rhizome. It is a perennial herb, similar in appearance to ginger. It has been used and cultivated in India since antiquity, being indigenous to southern Asia. Turmeric is a very popular Indian spice, medicine, and dye plant and is an important part of religious ceremonies in Hindu households. In 1950, there were over 100,000 acres of this herb in cultivation, according to one estimate (Wealth of India, 1950). It was introduced to China early on and was written of in the *Tang Pen Tsao* (1578) for its beneficial effects on the liver and digestion.

RELATED MEDICINAL SPECIES — Many of the species in the genus are used for flavoring food and as medicine, including *Curcuma aeruginosa* Roxb., used from Burma to Java and Indo-China as a medicine for colic; and *C. aromatica* Salisb., used in India and China as a stomachic and carminative (Perry, 1980). *Curcuma zedoary* is zedoary, widely used in India and China as a digestive and liver herb and as a condiment.

ENERGY, TASTE, CONSTITUTIONAL PROPERTIES — In Ayurveda, turmeric or *haridra* is considered a bitter drug, alleviating excess kapha. In TCM it is usually described as acrid, bitter, and warm

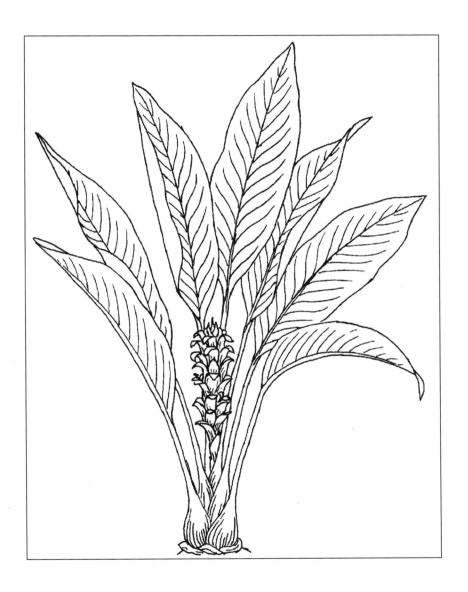

Turmeric — *Curcuma longa L.*

and is said to enter the spleen, stomach, and liver meridians. Like ginger, it is used to invigorate the blood and remove deficiency cold. Bensky and Gamble report that it "moves the Qi and alleviates pain: used for Stagnant Qi generated epigastric and abdominal pain. It also dispels Wind." In TEM, ginger was used in preference to turmeric. Turmeric is a *specific* and *protective* herb.

CONTRAINDICATIONS — Bensky and Gamble caution that turmeric is contraindicated "in cases of Deficient Blood without Stagnant Qi or Congealed Blood." Yeung (1985) lists pregnancy and anemia as contraindicated conditions.

CHEMICAL CONSTITUENTS AND PHYSIOLOGICAL ACTIVITIES — Turmeric contains a mixture of phenolic compounds called *curcumin*, and a volatile oil with turmerone and zingiberene; cineole and other monoterpenes; starch; protein; and high amounts of vitamin A and other vitamins.

The essential oil has proven stimulating effects on the gallbladder (perhaps due to the p-tolylmehyl carbinol) and also stimulates the liver to produce more bile and regulate its viscosity. Modern research also shows that the herb possesses anti—inflammatory and strong liver-protecting properties.

SPECIFIC USES — This herb is useful as a condiment to improve digestive function, especially in meals with many kinds of food combinations. It is also helpful for diarrhea and cold and weak digestive tone; environmental toxin poisoning; heavy metal poisoning; hepatitis; and to help remove pains in the liver and stomach. New studies show that zedoary root may be one of the best herbs for killing amoebae such as *Entamoeba histolytic*—a major cause of amoebic dysentery (Ansari, 1991).

PREPARATIONS, FORMULAS, AND DOSES — Turmeric can be purchased in powder form to be used for cooking or encapsulating, but I prefer the whole rhizome or at least the cut and sifted herb. This herb is included in many Ayurvedic patent formulas, and, increasingly, in Western formulas both in Europe and the United States for liver and digestive ailments. The average therapeutic dose of the tincture is 1 - 3 dropperfuls 2 to 3 times daily in tea or warm water. Of the powdered extract, take 60 to 300 mg. Of the powder, take 0.5 to 1.5 grams 2-3 times daily.

NOTES — Turmeric is recognizable as a major flavor component of many Indian dishes. The herb's good taste, coupled with its ability to aid digestion of fatty foods and starch/protein combinations, has made it increasingly popular in this country.

APPENDIX A
RESOURCES

Health Centers

Kripalu Institute P.O. Box 793, Lenox, MA 01240; (413) 637-3280

Ann Wigmore Foundation 196 Commonwealth Ave., Boston, MA 02116; (800) 966-9525

The Kushi Institute P.O. Box 7, Becket, MA 01223; (413) 623-5741

Esalen Institute, Big Sur, CA ; (408) 667-3000

Live Plants

Richter's Goodwood, Ontario, Canada LOC1AO; (416) 640-6677

Taylor's Herb Garden 1535 Lone Oak Rd., Vista, CA 92084; (704) 683-2014

Sandy Mush Herbs Surrett Cove Rd.; Leicester, NC 28748-9622; (704) 683-2014; send $4 for catalogue

Chinese Herb Dealers (mail order)

Mayway 622 Broadway, SF, CA 94133; (415) 788-3646

Western Herb Dealers (mail order)

Blessed Herbs: Rte. 5, Box 1042, Ava, MO 65608; (417) 683-5721

Inspiring Books

Bernie Siegel
Love, Medicine and Miracles; Peace, Love and Healing.

Louise Hay

Love Your Body; Heal Your Body; You Can Heal Your Life

Svevo Brooks
The Art of Good Living

Vivekenanda.
Karma Yoga, others

Paul Bragg
The Miracle of Fasting, *Healthy Eating Without Confusion*; many
other books.

Bernard Jensen
Nature Has a Remedy; Tissue Cleansing Through Bowel Management;
many other books.

Kristina Turner
The *Self-Healing Cookbook.*

René Dubos
Mirage of Health, any other books.

J. Krishnamurti
any books.

Journals

HerbalGram: P.O. Box 201660, Austin, TX 78720

The American Herb Assn. Quarterly Newsletter: P.O. Box 353,
Rescue, CA 95672

Medical Herbalism: P.O. Box 33080, Portland, OR 97233

REFERENCES

General References

Anon. 1827. *Sure Methods of Improving Health, and Prolonging Life.* London: Simpkin and Marshall.

Cheung, C.S. 1983. The Liver and Gall Bladder. *J. Am. Col. Trad. Ch. Med.* 2:30.

Davis, B.O., Holtz, N. & J.C. Davis. 1985. *Conceptual Human Physiology.* Columbus: Charles E. Merrill Pub. Co.

Farnsworth, N.R. 1980. "Botanical Sources of Fertility Regulating Agents: Chemistry and Pharmacology" in *Progress in Hormone Biochemistry and Pharmacology*, v. 1, Eden Press, Lancaster, England.

Gandhi, M.K. 1949. *Diet and Diet Reform.* Ahmedabad: Navajivan Pub. House.

Kellogg, J.H. 1916. *Colon Hygiene.* Battle Creek: Good Health Publishing Co.

Levine, S.A. & P.M. Kidd. 1985. *Antioxidant Adaptation.* San Leandro, CA: Biocurrents Division, Allergy Research Group.

MacFadden, B. 1929. *Digestive Troubles.* New York: Macfadden Publications, Inc.

Merck & Co. 1982. *The Merck Manual*, 14th ed. Rahway, IN: Merck.

Quintanilha, A. (ed.). 1988. *Reactive Oxygen Species in Chemistry, Biology, and Medicine.* New York: Plenum Press.

Reed, G. (ed.). 1983. *Food and Feed Production with Microorganisms.* Weinheim: Verlag Chemie. From *Biotechnology (A Comprehensive Treatise in 8 Volumes)*, v. 5, H.-J. Rehm and G. Reed, eds.

Reynolds, E.S. 1980. *Liver and Biliary Tree* in Systemic Reactions to

Injury by Environmental Agents.

Reynolds, E.S. 1980. *Free-Radical Damage in Liver* in Free Radicals in Biology, v. IV, p. 49. New York: Academic Press.

Rose, RC, et al. 1986. Transport and Metabolism of Vitamins. *Federation Proceedings* 45:30.

Salunkhe D.K., et al. (date missing). Anticancer Agents of Plant Origin, CRC Critical Reviews in Plant Sciences; Vol. 1, Issue 3, p. 218.

Tepperman, J. 1980. *Metabolic and Endocrine Physiology*, 4th ed. Chicago: Year Book Medical Publishers, Inc.

Tierra, M. 1988. *Planetary Herbology*. Santa Fe: Lotus Press.

Tilden, J.H. 1916-7. *Philosophy of Health*, v. 17. Denver: Tilden.

Tortora, G.J. 1980. *Principles of Human Anatomy*. New York: Harper & Row.

Vander, A.J., Sherman, J.H., & D.S. Luciano. 1980. *Human Physiology*. New York: McGraw-Hill Book Co.

Vogel, A. (1962). *The Liver*, Bioforce-Verlag Teufen, Switzerland.

Walker, N.W. 1979. *Colon Health*. Phoenix: O. Sullivan Woodside & Co.

Yanchi, L. 1988. *The Essential Book of Traditional Chinese Medicine*. New York: Columbia University Press..

References for Probiotic Chapter (Chapter 4)

Symposium: "Probiotics: The Friendly Bacteria." February 15, 1992, Dallas, Texas. Sponsored by the South Western Health Organization. Speakers: Silvano Arnoldo, George Weber, Randolph Porubcan, Jarrow Rogovin, Anthony Almada, Robert Sellars, S.K. Dash, Khem Shahani. Selected parts of the above presenters' talks was paraphrased for the "Using Probiotic Supplements" section. Tapes of the conference are available through Tree Farm Communications, 23703 NE 4th St., Redmond, WA 98053.

Bailey, P. 1992. Personal Communication.

Recommended Reading

Chaitow, L. & N. Trenev. 1990. *Probiotics.* Wellingborough, England: Thorson's Publishing Group.

Drasar, B.S. and M.J. Hill. 1974. *Human Intestinal Flora.* London: Academic Press.

Hentges, D.J., ed. 1983. *Human Intestinal Microflora in Health and Disease.* New York: Academic Press.

Hesseltine, C.W. & H.L. Wang. 1986. *Indigenous Fermented Food of Non-Western Origin.* Berllin: J. Cramer.

Kurmann, J.A., J.L. Rasic, and M. Kroger. 1992. *Encyclopedia of Fermented Fresh Milk Products.* New York: Van Nostrand Reinhold.

Metchnikoff, E. 1904. *The Nature of Man.* London: William Heinemann, p. 253.

Rasic, J.L., and J.A. Kuirssann. (1983). *Bifidobacteria and their Role.* Boston: Birkhaüser Verlag.

Steinkraus, K.H., et al., ed. 1983. *Handbook of Indigenous Fermented Foods.* New York: Marcel Dekker, Inc.

General References (Probiotics)

Anon. 1984. Lactobacillus feeding alters human colonic bacterial enzyme activities. *Nutr. Rev.* 42:374-376.

Anon. 1991. Infectious Disease News. Hydrogen Peroxide Producing Organisms Toxic To Vaginal Bacteria. *Infectious Disease News.* Aug. 8: 5. From CPC 1:315.

Anon. 1991. Premature Birth and Vaginal Bacteria. *CP News.* 1(2):7.

Anon. 1991. Vaginitis and Hydrogen Peroxide. *CP News.* 1(2):7.

Abrams, G.D. 1983. Impact of the Intestinal Microflora on Intestinal

Structure and Function. Hentges (*Human Intestinal Micro-flora...*) p.291.

Abrosimova, N.A., et al. 1989. Creating the optimal microecology of the intestines in premature newborn infants with the sour-milk mixture "biphilin". *Pediatriia.* (3):30-33.

Alm, L. 1983. The effect of Lactobacillus acidophilus administration upon the survival of Salmonella in randomly selected human carriers. *Prog. Food Nutr. Sci.* 7:13-17.

Alm, L., et al. 1983. The Effect of Acidophilus milk in the treatment of constipation in hospitalised geriatric patients. *XV Symp. Swed. Nutr. Found:*131-138.

Alm. L. 1984. Acidophilus milk for therapy in gastrointestinal disorders. *Nahrung.* 28:683-684.

Ayebo, A.D., et al. 1980. Effect of ingesting Lactobacillus acidophi-lus milk upon fecal flora and enzyme activity in humans. *Milchwissenschaft.* 35:730-733.

Bellomo, G., et al. 1980. A controlled double-blind study of S.F.68 strain as a new biological preparation for the treatment of diarrhoea in pediatrics. *Current Therapeutic Research.* 28:927-936.

Benno, Y., et al. 1984. The intestinal microflora of infants: compo-sition of fecal flora in breast-fed and bottle-fed infants. *Microbiol. Immunol.* 28:975-986.

Borgia, M., et al. 1982. A controlled clinical study on Streptococcus faecium preparation for the prevention of side reactions during long-term antibiotic treatments. *Current Therapeutic Research.* 31:265-271.

Bornside, G.H. 1978. Stability of human fecal flora. *The American Journal of Clinical Nutrition.* 31:S14-S144.

Burkitt, D.P. 1978. Colonic-rectal cancer: fiber and other dietary factors. *The American Journal of Clinical Nutrition.* 31:S58-S64.

Burkitt, D.P. 1978. Workshop V—Fiber and cancer. Summary and recommendations. *The American Journal of Clinical Nutrition.* 31:S213-S215.

Butler, B.C., and J.W. Beakley. 1960. Bacterial flora in vaginitis. *Am.*

J. Obst. & Gynec. 79:432-440.

Camarri, E., et al. 1981. A double-blind comparison of two different treatments for acute enteritis in adults. *Chemotherapy.* 27:466-470.

Chernyshova, L.I. 1989. Effects of dysbacteriosis and impairment of immunity formation in the early neonatal period on morbidity of children during the 1st year of life and ways of its reduction. *Pediatriia.* (6):24-29.

Clements, M.L., et al.1984. Exogenous lactobacilli fed to man - their fate and ability to prevent diarrheal disease.*J. Natl. Cancer Inst.*73:689-695.

Colle, R. and T. Ceschia. 1989. Oral bacteriotherapy with *Bifidobacterium bifidum* and *Lactobacillus acidophilus* in cirrhotic patients. *Clin. Ter.* 131:397-402.

Collins,E.B. and P. Hardt. 1980. Inhibition of *Candida albicans* by *Lactobacillus acidophilus. J. Dairy Sci.* 63:830-832.

Conway, P.L., et al. 1987. Survival of lactic acid bacteria in the human stomach and adhesion to intestinal cells. *J. Dairy Sci.* 70(1):1-12.

Cummings, J.H. 1983. Fermentation in the human large intestine: evidence and implications for health. *The Lancet.* May 28:1206-1208.

Cummings, J.H. 1983. Dietary fibre and the intestinal microflora. *XV Symp. Swed. Nutr. Found.*: 77-84.

Cummings, J.H., et al. 1979. The effect of meat protein and dietary fiber on colonic function nd metabolism. II. Bacterial metabolites in feces in urine. *The American Journal of Clinical Nutrition.* 32:2094-2101.

Darby, W.J. 1979. *The Nutrient Contributions of Fermented Beverages.* Gastineau, p.61.

Davenport, H.W. 1982. *Physiology of the Digestive Tract*, 5th edition. Chicago: Year Book Medical Publishers.

Drasar, B.S. and M.J. Hill. 1974. *Human Intestinal Flora.* London: Academic Press.

Drasar, B.S., et al. 1986. Diet and faecal flora in three dietary groups in rural northern Nigeria. *J. Hyg., Camb.* 96:59-65.

Eastwood, M.A. 1978. Fiber in the gastrointestinal tract. *The American Journal of Clinical Nutrition.* 31:S30-S32.

Ehle, F.R., et al. 1981. Dietary fibers on fermemtation in the human. *J. Nutr.* 112:158-166.

Ensminger, A.H., et al. 1983. *Foods and Nutrition Encyclopedia.* Clovis, CA: Pegus Press.

Erasmus, U. 1986. *Fats and Oils.* Burnaby BC: Alive Books.

Finegold, S.M. and V.L. Sutter. 1978. Fecal flora in different populations, with special reference to diet. *The American Journal of Clinical Nutrition.* 31:S116-S122.

Fleming, L. L., et al. 1986. Digestion and absorption of fiber carbohydrate in the colon. *The American Journal of Gastroenterology.* 81(7): 507-510.

Fredricsson, B., et al. 1989. Bacterial vaginosis is not a simple ecololgical disorder. *Gynecol. Obstet. Invest.* 28:156-160.

Friedlander, A., et al. 1986. *Lactobacillus acidophillus* and vitamin B complex in the treatment of vaginal infection. *Panminerva Medica.* 28:51-53.

Friedlander, A., et al.1986. *Lactobacillus acidophillus* and vitamin B complex in the treatment of vaginal infection. *Panminerva Med.* 28(1):51-53.

Friis-Moller, A. and H. Hey. 1983. Colonization of the intestinal canal with a *Streptococcus faecium* preparation (Paraghurt). *Current Therapeutic Research.* 33:807-815.

Fuller, R., et al. 1981. Attachment of *Streptococcus faecium* to the duodenal epithelium of the chicken and its importance in colonization of the small intestine. *Applied and Environmental Microbiology.* 41:1433-1441.

Gastineau, C.F., et al., ed. 1979. *Fermented Food Beverages In Nutrition.* New York: Academic Press.

Gilbert, J.P., et al. 1983. Viricidal effects of *Lactobacillus* and yeast fermentation. *Appl. Environ. Microbiol.* 46:452-458.

Gilliland, S.E. and D.K. Walker. 1990. Factors to consider when selecting a culture of *Lactobacillus acidophilus* as a dietary adjunct to produce a hypocholesterolemic effect in humans. *J. Dairy Sci.* 73:905-911.

Goldin, B., et al. 1978. Influence of diet and age on fecal bacterial enzymes. *The American Journal of Clinical Nutiriton.* 31:S136-S140.

Goldin, B.R. and S.L. Gorbach. 1984a. The effect of milk and lactobacillus feeding on human intestinal bacterial enzyme activity. *The American Journal of Clinical Nutrition.* 39:756-761.

Goldin, B.R., and S.L. Gorbach. 1984b. Alterations of the intestinal microflora by diet, oral antibiotics, and Lactobacillus: decreased production of free amines from aromatic nitro compounds, azo dyes, and gluronides. *Microbiologica.* 7:331-339.

Gonzalez, S.N., et al.1983. Oral bacteriotheraphy with *Bifidobacterium bifidum* and *Lactobacillus acidophilus* in cirrhotic patients. *Prog. Food Nutr. Sci.* 7:29-37.

Gorbach, S.L. 1986. Bengt E. Gustfsson memorial lecture. Function of the normal human microflora. *Scand. J. Infect. Dis Suppl.* 49:17-30.

Goto, T. et al. 1988. Induction of interferon by Lactobacillus. *Kansenshogaku Zasshi.* 62(12):1105-1110.

Graf, W. 1983. Studies on the Therapeutic properties of acidophilus milk. *XV Symp. Swed. Nutr. Found*: 119-120.

Gregori, G., et al. 1985. Use of oral bacteria therapy in childhood during acute enteritis and functional chronic diarrhea. Clinical experience. *Acta Biomed. Ateneo Parmense.* 56:23-26.

Gustafsson, B.E. 1983. Introduction to the ecology of the intestinal microflora and its general characteristics. *XV Symp.Swed. Nutr. Found:11-15.*

Marild, S., et al. 1990. Urinary Tract Infection; Breast Feeding. *Clinical Pearls in Nutrition and Preventive Medicine.* 347.

Hanson, L.Å, et al. 1983. The gut and the immune response. *XV Symp Swed. Nutr Found.:63-67.*

Heneghan, J.B. 1973, ed. *International Symposium on Germfree Research* (4th, 1972). New York: Academic Press.

Hentges, D.J. 1986. The protective function of the indigenous intestinal flora. *Pediatric Infectious Disease.* 5(1):S17-S20.

Hentges, D.J., ed. 1983. *Human Intestinal Microflora in Health and Disease.* New York: Academic Press.

Hill, M.J., ed. 1986. *Microbial Metabolism in the Digestive Tract.* Florida: CRC Press.

Hooker, K.D. and J.T. DiPiro. 1988. Effect of antimicrobial therapy on bowel flora. *Clinical Pharmacy.* 7:878-888.

Hungate, E. 1978. Bacterial ecology in the small intestine. *The American Journal of Clinical Nutrition.* 31:S125-S127.

Kim, H.S. 1983. *Lactobacillus acidophilus* as a dietary adjunct for milk to aid lactose digestion in humans. *J. Dairy Sci.* 66:959-966.

Kritchevsky, D. 1978. Workshop IV-Fiber, lipids, and cardiovascular disease. Summary and recommendations. *The American Journal of Clinical Nutrition.* 31:S190.

Lewenstein. A., et al. 1979. Biological properties of SF 68, a new approach for the treatment of diarrheal diseases. *Current Therapeutic Research.* 26:967-981.

Lidbeck, A., et al. 1987. Impact of *Lactobacillus acidophilus* supplements on the human oropharyngeal and intestinal microflora. *Scand. J. Infect. Dis.* 19:531-537.

Lidbeck, A., et al. 1988. Impact of Lactobacillus acidophilus on the normal intestinal microflora ater administration of two antimicrobial agents. *Infection.* 16:329-336.

Macdonald,I.A., et al. 1978. Fecal hydroxysteroid dehydrogenase activities in vegetarian Seventh-Day Adventists, control subjects, and bowel cancer patients. *The Americal Journal of Clinical Nutrition.* 31:S233-S238.

Marchetti, F., et al. 1987. Efficacy of regulators of the intestinal bacterial flora in the therapy of acne vulgaris. *Clin. Ter.* 122(5):339-343.

Marteau, P., et al. 1990. Effect of chronic ingestion of a fermented dairy product containing *Lactobacillus acidophilus* and *Bifidobacterium bifidum* on metabolic activities of the colonic flora in humans. *Am. J. Clin. Nur.* 52:685-688.

McDonough, F.E., et al. 1987. Modification of sweet acidophilus milk to improve utilization by lactose-intolerant persons. *Am. J. Clin. Nutr.* 45(3):570-574.

McGroarty, J.A. and G. Reid. 1988. Detection of a Lactobacillus substance that inhibits Escherichia coli. *Can. J. Microbiol.* 34:974-978.

Midtvedt, A.C., et al. 1988. Development of five metabolic activities associated with the intestinal microflora of healthy infants. *Journal of Pediatric Gastroenterology and Nutrition.* 7:559-567.

Midtvedt, T. 1987. Intestinal bacteria and rheumatic disease. *Scand. J. Rheumatology.* Suppl. 64:49-54.

Moshchich, P.S., et al. 1989. Prevention of dysbacteriosis in the early neonatal period using a pure culture of acidophillic bacteria. *Pediatriia.* (3)25-30.

Nord, C.E., et al. 1984. Impact of antimicrobial agents on the gastrointestinal microflora and the risk of infections. *The American Journal of Medicine.* 76:99-106.

Nordbring, F. 1983. Antibiotics in human therapy. *XV Symp. Swed. Nutr. Found.:* 87-92.

Perdigon, G., et al. 1988. Adjuvant activity of lactic bacteria: perspectives for its use in oral vaccines. *Rev.Argent Microbiol.* 20(3):141-146.

Peridgon, G., et al. 1988. Systemic augmentation of the immune response in mice by feeding fermented milks with *Lactobacillus casei* and *Lactobacillus acidophilus. Immunology.* 63(1):17-23.

Pettersson,L., et al. 1983. Survival of *Lactobacillus acidophilus* NCDO 1748 in the human gastrointestinal tract 1. Incubation with gastric juice in vitro. *XV Symp. Swed. Nutr. Found:* 1123-125.

Pettersson, L. et al. 1983. Survival of Lactobacillus acidophilus NCDO 1748 in the human gastrointestinal tract 2. Ability to pass the stomach and intestine in vivo. *XV Symp. Swed. Nutr. Found:* 127-130.

Pradham, A. and M.K. Majumdar. 1986. Metabolism of some drugs by intestinal Lactobacilli and their toxicological considerations. *Acta Pharmacol. et Toxicol.* 58:11-15.

Rasic, J.L., and J.A. Kuirssann. 1983. *Bifidobacteria and their Role.* Boston: Birkhaüser Verlag.

Reddy, G.V., et al. 1983. Natural antibiotic activity of *Lactobacillus acidophilus* and *bulgaraicus*. *Cultured Dairy Products Journal*.

Reid, G., et al. 1985. Prevention of urinary tract infection in rats with an indigenous *lactobacillus casei* strain. *Infection and Immunity*. 49:320-324.

Salminen, E., et al. 1988. Preservation of intestinal integrity during radiotherapy using live *Lactobacillus acidophilus* cultures. *Clin. Radiol.* 39(4):435-437.

Salyers, A.A. 1983. Metabolic activities of intestinal bacteria. *XV Symp.Swed. Nutr. Found.*: 35-43.

Sandstead, H.H., et al. 1978. Influence of dietary fiber on trace element balance. *The American Journal of Clinical Nutrition*. 31:S180-S184.

Sarra, P.G., et al. 1989. Colonization of a human intestine by four different genotypes of *Lactobacillus acidophilus*. *Gynecol. Obstet. Invest.* 28:156-160.

Savage, D.C. 1983. Microbial ecology of the gastrointestinal tract. *XV Symp. Swed. Nutr. Found.*: 17-23.

Savaiano, D. A., et al. 1984. Lactose malabsorption from yogurt, pasteurized yogurt, sweet Acidophilus milk, and cultured milk in lactase-deficient individuals. *The American Journal of Clinical Nurition*. 40:1219-1223.

Shahani, K.M. and A.D. Ayebo. 1980. Role of dietary lactobacilli in gastrointestinal microecology. *The American Journal of Clinical Nutrition*. 33: 2448-2457.

Shahani, K.M. 1983. Nutritional impact of Lactobacillic fermented foods.*XV Symp. Swed. Nutr. Found:* 103-109.

Southgate, T. 1978. Dietary fiber: analysis and food sources. *The American Journal of Clinical Nutrition*. 31:S107-S110.

Speck, M.L. 1983. *Lactobacilli* as dietary supplements and manifestations of their functions in the intestine. *XV Symp. Swed. Nutr. Found.*: 93-97

Steinkraus, K.H., et al., eds. 1983. *Handbook of Indigenous Fermented Foods*. New York: Marcel Dekker, Inc.

Tabaqchali, S. et al. 1986. Bacterial flora and intestinal chronic diseases. *Ann. Ist. Super. Sanita*. 22(3): 921-932.

Tannock, G.W. 1983. Effect of dietary and environmental stress on the gastrointestinal microbiota. Hentges, p. 517.

Todhunter, E. N. 1979. *A Historical Perspective on Fermentation Biochemistry and Nutrition*. Gastineau, p.83.

van der Weiden, R.M., et al. 1990. Treatment failure in trichomoniasis and persistence of the parasite after *Lactobacillus* immunotherapy; two case report. *Eur. J. Obstet. Gynecol. Reprod. Biol.* 34:171-178.

Vincent, J.G., et al. 1959. Antibacterial activity associated with *Lactobacillus acidophilus*. 78:477-484.

Visek, W.J. 1978. Diet and cell growth modulation by ammonia. *The American Journal of Clinical Nutrition*. 31:S216-S220.

Yoshioka, H., et al. 1983. Development and differences of intestinal flora in the neonatal period in breast-fed and bottle-fed infants. *Pediatrics*.72:317-321.

Young. G., et al. 1956. Interactions of oral strains of *Candida albicans* and *Lactobacilli*. *J. Bact.* 72:525-529.

References for Herbal

References Consulted for History of Use

Alleyne, J. 1733. *A New English Dispensatory*. London: Tho. Astley.

Cockayne, O. 1864. *Leechdoms, Wortcunning, and Starcraft.* London: Longman, Green, Longman, Roberts, and Green.

Culpeper, N. 1650. *A Physical Directory: or a Translation of the Dispensatory made by the Colledge of Physitians of London.* London: Peter Cole.

Dierbach, J.H. 1824. *Die Arzneimittel des Hippokrates.* Heidelberg: Neue Akademische Buchhandlung von Karl Groos. Translation by Christopher Hobbs and Shanti Coble.

Dodoens, R. 1586. *A New Herball, or Historie of Plants.* London: Ninian Newton.

Dragendorff, G. 1898. *Die Heilpflanzen der Verschiedenen Völker und Zeiten.* Stuttgart: Verlag von Ferdinand Enke.

Farnsworth, N.R., et al. 1957-1974. *The Lynn Index.* Chicago: College of Pharmacy, University of Illinois at the Medical Center.

Gerard, J. & Johnson, T. (ed.). 1633. *The Herbal or General History of Plants.* Reprinted by Dover Publications, New York (1975).

Felter, H.W. & J.U. Lloyd. 1898. *King's American Dispensatory.* Cincinnati: The Ohio Valley Co.

Gunther, R.T. 1933. *The Greek Herbal of Dioscorides.* New York: Hafner Pub. Co. (1968).

Hort, A.F., tr. 1948. *Theophrastus Enquiry into Plants.* Cambridge: Harvard University Press.

Jones, W.H.S. 1956. Pliny: *Natural History.* Cambridge: Harvard University Press.

Levey, M. 1966. *The Medical Formulary or Aqrabadhin of Al-Kindi. Madison: The University of Wisconsin Press.*

Lewis, W. 1791. *An Experimental History of the Materia Medica.* London: J. Johnson.

Madaus, G. 1938. *Handbook of Biological Medicine.* Reprinted by George Olms Verlag, NY (1976).

Pereira, J. 1843. *The Elements of Materia Medica and Therapeutics,* 1st American edition from the 2nd London, with notes and additions by J. Carson. Philadelphia: Lea & Blanchard.

Pickering, C. 1879. *Chronological History of Plants.* Boston: Little, Brown & Co.

Pughe, J., tr. & J. Williams, ed. 1861. *The Physicians of Myddvai.* London: Longman & Co.

References for Ayurveda

Ainslie, W. 1826. *Materia Medica*. London: Longman, Rees, Orme, Brown and Green. Reprinted by Periodical Expert Book Agency, Delhi (1979).

Chadha, Y.R., chief ed. 1952-88. *The Wealth of India* (Raw Materials), 11 vols. New Delhi: Publications and Information Directorate, CSIR.

Dash, V.B. & L. Kashyap. 1987 (1980). *Materia Medica of Ayurveda*. New Delhi: Concept Publishing Company.

Dash, V.B. & A.M.M. Junius. 1988. *A Handbook of Ayurveda*. New Delhi: Concept Publishing Co.

Dymock, W. 1890. *Pharmacographia Indica*. Bombay: Education Society's Press.

References for Traditional Chinese Medicine

Bensky, D. & A. Gamble. 1986. *Chinese Herbal Medicine, Materia Medica*. Seattle: Eastland Press.

Bretschneider, E. 1895. *Botanicon Sinicum*. Hong Kong: Kelly & Walsh, Ltd.

Chang, H.-M. & P.P.-H. But. 1986. *Pharmacology and Applications of Chinese Materia Medica*, 2 volumes. Philadelphia: World Scientific.

Chang, H.M., et al. 1985. *Advances in Chinese Medicinal Materials Research*. Philadelphia: World Press.

Hooper, D. 1929 (1969). On Chinese Medicine: Drugs of Chinese Pharmacies in Malaya. *The Gardens' Bulletin, Straits Settlements* 6:165.

Hsu, H.-Y. 1980. *How to Treat Yourself with Chinese Herbs*. Los

Angeles: Oriental Healing Arts Institute.

Hsu, H.-Y., et al. 1986. *Oriental Materia Medica, a concise guide.* Long Beach, CA: Oriental Healing Arts Institute.

Maciocia. 1989. *The Foundations of Chinese Medicine.* Singapore: Churchill Livingstone.

National Academy of Sciences. 1975. *Herbal Pharmacology in the People's Republic of China.* Washington: National Academy of Sciences.

Zhicen, L., et al. (eds.). 1987. *Colour Atlas of Chinese Traditional Drugs,* v. 1. Beijing: Science Press.

Perry, L.M. 1980. Medicinal Plants of East and Southeast Asia. Cambridge: The MIT Press.

Smith, F.P. & G.A. Stuart. 1973. *Chinese Medicinal Herbs.* San Francisco: Georgetown Press.

Steward, A.N. 1958. *Manual of Vascular Plants of the Lower Yangtze Valley, China.* Corvalis, OR: Oregon State University.

Yeung, H.-C. 1985. *Handbook of Chinese Herbs and Formulas,* v. 1. Los Angeles: Institute of Chinese Medicine.

Veith, I. 1972. *The Yellow Emperor's Classic of Internal Medicine.* Berkeley: University of California Press.

References for Bitters Section

Maiwald, L. 1987. Bitterstoffe. *Zeitschrift für Phytotherapie* 8: 186-88.

References for Fasting Section

Bragg, P.C. 1976. *The Miracle of Fasting.* Desert Hot Springs: Health Science.

Ehret, A. 1971. *Rational Fasting for Physical, Mental and Spiritual Rejuvenation.* Beaumont, CA: Ehret Literature Publishing Co.

Kellog, J.H. 1927. *The New Dietetics.* Battle Creek: The Modern Medicine Publishing Co.

Krok, M. 1967. *Fruit the Food and Medicine for Man.* Westville, Natal, South Africa: Essence of Health.

Lindlahr, H. 1937. *Nature Cure.* Poona, India: Dr. M.B. Godbole.

Macfadden, B. & F. Oswald. [n.d.]. *Macfadden's Fasting, Hydropathy and Exercise.* London: Bernarr Macfadden.

Macfadden, B. 1924. *Fasting for Health.* New York: Macfadden Pub.

McCoy, F. 1926. *The Fast Way to Health.* Los Angeles: McCoy Publications, Inc.

McFadden, B. & Fleming, W.F. (ed.). 1909. *Physical Culture Classics* in four volumes. New York J.F. Tapley Co.

General Herbal References

Ansari, M.H. & S. Ahmad. 1991. "Screening of some Medicinal Plants for Antiamoebic Action. *Fitoterapiea* 62: 171-5.

Benoit, P.S., et al. 1976. t.m. *Lloydia* 39: 160.

Cazin, F.-J. 1886. *Plantes Médicinales.* Paris: Asselin & Houzeau.

Felter, H.W. & J.U. Lloyd. 1898. *King's American Dispensatory.* Cincinnati: The Ohio Valley Co.

Hikino, H. 1986. Antihepatotoxic Actions of *Allium sativum* Bulbs. *Planta Medica* 52:163.

Iwagawa, T. , et al. 1985. *Kagoshima Daigaku Rigakubu Kiyo.* 18: 49-52. Through CA111001.

Kaptchuk, T.J. 1983. *The Web That Has no Weaver.* NY: Congdon & Weed.

Kimura Y, et al. 1984. Studies on Scutellariae Radix; IX-New Component Inhibiting Lipid Peroxidation in Rat Liver, *Planta Medica* 50:290.

Kimura Y, et al. 1985. Effects of Extracts of Leaves of Artemisia Species....on Lipid Metabolic Injury in Rats Fed Peroxidized Oil. *Chem. Pharm. Bull.* 33:2028-2034.

Kiso, Y., et al. 1985. Mechanism of Antihepatoxic Activity of Wuweisisu C and Gomisin A. *Planta Medica* 51:331-334.

Kiso, Y., et al. 1984. Antihepatotoxic Principles of Artemisia capillaris Buds. *Planta Medica* 50:81.

Leung, A.Y. 1980. *Encyclopedia of Natural Ingredients.* New York: John Wiley & Sons.

Lewis, W. 1791. *An Experimental History of the Materia Medica.* London: J. Johnson.

List, P.H. and L. Hörhammer. 1973. *Hagers Handbuch der Pharmazeutischen Praxis,* 7 vols. New York: Springer-Verlag.

Maeda, S., et al. 1985. Effects of Gomisin A on Liver Functions in Hepatotoxic Chemicals-Treated Rats. *Japan J. Pharmacol.* 38:347-353.

Moore, M. 1979. *Medicinal Plants of the Mountain West.* Santa Fe: Museum of New Mexico Press.

Salbe, A.D. and L.F. Bjeldanes. 1985. The Effects of Dietary Brussel Sprouts and Schizandra chinensis on the Xenobiotic-Metabolizing Enzymes of the Rat Small Intestines. *Food Chem Toxic* 23:57.

Tiantong B., et al. 1980. A Comparison of the Pharmacologic Actions of 7 Constituents Isolated From Fructus Schizandrae, *Chinese Med. J.* 93:41-47.

Index

A

Abdominal pain
  turmeric for 288
Abscess
  dandelion for 253
Acidophilus
  benefits of 97–99
  benefits, summary 98–99
  survival rate 99
Acne. *See* Digestive ailments,
    programs for: skin disorders
    (acne, psoriasis)
  burdock for 229
  chicory for 240
  dietary recommendations
    for 198
  gentian for 262
  herbal recommendations
    for 198–199
Addictions
  dietary recommendations
    for 205
  gentian for 262
  herbal recommendations
    for 205
Adrenals, weakened
  schisandra for 285
Aduki beans 107
Air, fresh- bath 151
Almond seed 110
Aloe 130
Amaranth
  nutritional value of 49

Amino acids 58
Amla 132
Ammonia
  protection from 69
Amoebic dysentery
  turmeric for 288
Anemia
  bitters, improvement with 120
Angelica 115, 122, 126, 128,
    210–214
  bitters and 213
Angostura 115
Anorexia
  blessed thistle for 223
Anti-spasmodics 110
Antibiotic treatment
  probiotic supplements for 89–
    91
Antibiotics
  side effects of 71–73
  side effects, ways to mini-
    mize 75–76
Antiinflammatory herbs
  citrus 243–244
Appendicitis 195
  dandelion for 254
Appetite, loss of
  berberis for 217
  bupleurum and cinnamon
    formula for 226
Appetite, poor
  bitters, improvement
    with 120, 262
  blessed thistle for 223

Caraway 110, 137
Cardamon 115
Cascara 122, 126, 130, 158,
    230–233
  contraindications 230
  use of 232
Catechin 58
Cathartics 129–130
Catnip 170
Cayenne 130
Celandine 125
Centaury 122, 125
Chamomile 110, 136–137, 170
Chaparral 124, 126, 141
Chebulic myrobalan 132
Chickweed
  nutritional value of 49
Chicory 50, 125, 158, 237–
    240
  contraindications 239–240
Chicory greens
  food use of 237
Children and infants
  probiotic programs for 90
Chlorella 107
Chlorine
  effect on probiotics 88
Cholesterol 81–82
  lowering effect of
      probiotics 70
  lowering with fiber 155
Cholesterol, high
  artichoke, beneficial effects
      of 216
  dandelion for 254
Cirrhosis. *See* Digestive ailments,
    programs for: hepatitis,
    cirrhosis
  bupleurum for 225

dan shen for 250
  milk thistle for 274
Citrus 241–245
Citrus peel, unripe 129
  contraindications of 241
Clay, bentonite
  uses 156
Cleansing 140
  blood purification 140–141
  bowel 152
    clay and pectin, with 155–
    156
  burdock for 229
  citrus for 243–244
  colonics 161
  enemas for 156–163
  fasting for 161
  gallbladder flush for 147–148
  kidneys, through 152
  liver flush for 145–147
  lymphatic 141–149
  red root for 283
  skin brushing, air baths
      for 150–151
  sweating therapy for 149–150
Cleavers 126, 144, 152
Codonopsis 107, 127
Coffee substitute
  chicory as 240
Coffee substitute, herbal 193
Coix 127, 128
Colic
  fringetree for 235
  ginger for 266
Colitis
  enemas, therapeutic for 160
  colitis 81
Colon inflammation
  enemas for 157

intestinal microflora, overview 61–62
introduction 60
protection from patho-
gens 66–67
regulation of mucus 71
supplements, commercial 88
amount, duration to take 92
form, best: powder, capsules,
etc. 91
questions, commonly
asked 89
reliability of 94–95
shelf life of 96
species, best 93–95
storage 95–96
when to take 92
toxins, protection from 69–70
vitamin synthesis and 69
probiotics
bacteriocins 86
Protein
proper amount 59
Protein assimilation, poor
berberis for 219
Psoriasis. *See* Digestive ailments,
programs for: skin disorders
(acne, psoriasis)
burdock for 229
milk thistle for 274
Psyllium 153
Psyllium, caution 154
Purslane
nutritional value of 49
Pussy paws 125

Q

Qi
regulation of by liver 32–33

Quassia 126
Quercetin 58

R

Red clover 141, 158
Red raspberry leaves 130
Red root 126, 144, 281–283
Rhamnosus, Lactobacillus ssp. casei
benefits of 100
Rhubarb 130
Rice sprouts 128
Root beer 229
Rosemary 123, 125
Rutin 58

S

Saffron 123
Sage 110
Sarsaparilla 141, 152
Sauerkraut 79–86
health benefits of 78
how to make 79–80
Schisandra 123, 124, 126, 284–
285
Selenium 58
Senna 70, 130
Silymarin
activity of 274
Skin damage
sun, from 151
Skullcap 124, 126
Slippery elm bark 110
Sour
therapeutic properties of 45
Spasms, digestive tract
ginger for 266
Spearmint 110
Spirulina 58, 107

Latin Index